Woman
Cancer
Sex

By Anne Katz, RN, PhD

Hygeia Media
An imprint of the Oncology Nursing Society
Pittsburgh, Pennsylvania

ONS Publishing Division
Publisher: Leonard Mafrica, MBA, CAE
Director, Commercial Publishing: Barbara Sigler, RN, MNEd
Managing Editor: Lisa M. George, BA
Technical Content Editor: Angela D. Klimaszewski, RN, MSN
Staff Editor: Amy Nicoletti, BA
Copy Editor: Laura Pinchot, BA
Graphic Designer: Dany Sjoen
Cover Design: Eric Marchetta

Woman Cancer Sex

Library of Congress Control Number: 20099923527

ISBN: 978-1-890504-80-9

Publisher's Note

This book is published by the Oncology Nursing Society (ONS). ONS neither represents nor guarantees that the practices described herein will, if followed, ensure safe and effective patient care. The recommendations contained in this book reflect ONS's judgment regarding the state of general knowledge and practice in the field as of the date of publication. The recommendations may not be appropriate for use in all circumstances. Those who use this book should make their own determinations regarding specific safe and appropriate patient-care practices, taking into account the personnel, equipment, and practices available at the hospital or other facility at which they are located. The editors and publisher cannot be held responsible for any liability incurred as a consequence from the use or application of any of the contents of this book. Figures and tables are used as examples only. They are not meant to be all-inclusive, nor do they represent endorsement of any particular institution by ONS. Mention of specific products and opinions related to those products do not indicate or imply endorsement by ONS. Web sites mentioned are provided for information only; the hosts are responsible for their own content and availability. Unless otherwise indicated, dollar amounts reflect U.S. dollars.

ONS publications are originally published in English. Publishers wishing to translate ONS publications must contact the ONS Publishing Division about licensing arrangements. ONS publications cannot be translated without obtaining written permission from ONS. (Individual tables and figures that are reprinted or adapted require additional permission from the original source.) Because translations from English may not always be accurate or precise, ONS disclaims any responsibility for inaccuracies in words or meaning that may occur as a result of the translation. Readers relying on precise information should check the original English version.

Printed in the United States of America

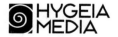

An imprint of the Oncology Nursing Society

For my Mouse
I carry you over my heart
To the nth

With grateful thanks to Jen Hellwig
for ideas

Contents

Preface

I have worked with many women over the years in my practice as a sexuality counselor for people with cancer. Some have had breast cancer; others have had cervical or uterine cancer. There have been women with lymphoma or leukemia, and some with melanoma, a skin cancer, that many healthcare providers never would have thought could have sexual problems related to its treatment.

All these women dealt with their illness and its consequences in different ways. All of them coped, but many were really sad at the changes in their lives and relationships. All of these women touched me and challenged me. I laughed with many (humor is a great healer) and cried with many, even if they didn't see the tears on the outside.

But those were the ones who were lucky enough or brave enough to get help from me, a professional who specializes in this area. What about the many millions of other women who have cancer or who have survived cancer and who have problems but are too far from a specialist to get help? Or who are too scared to ask their healthcare provider for a referral? What about the women who try to talk to their healthcare provider and are told that what they are going through has nothing to do with cancer or treatment?

This book is for these women and for the men and women who love them.

PART ONE

Understanding the Basics

Why is sex important to us as individuals and as couples? How do we become sexual beings, and what influences it? This introductory chapter will set the stage for the rest of the book by describing the anatomy of the sex organs and how things work.

CHAPTER 1

Introduction

Sex and sexuality are important aspects of life for women in the 21st century. We all are aware of ourselves as sexual beings, whether we express that with a partner or alone, frequently or infrequently, proudly or with conflicted feelings.

So what's the difference between sexuality and sexual functioning? *Sexuality* has been defined as the way we experience and express ourselves as sexual beings. This begins in infancy and persists through old age and is influenced by the norms of our families, communities, and society as a whole. It includes our awareness of ourselves as female and male and is an essential part of who we are and how we interact with others, irrespective of whether we actually engage in sexual activity or not. Our sexuality persists even when we're faced with challenges; it's not based in our breasts or genitalia but rather in our hearts, minds, and souls. We may feel pleasurable sensations in our genitals, but we experience those sensations in our heads and hearts, too. Part of our sexuality embraces how we seek out pleasure, intimacy, and connectedness with our partner, as well as how we experience erotic thoughts and feelings. Our sexual orientation, or with whom we choose to be sexual, is an intrinsic part of sexuality. For some of us, procreation or reproduction is the expression of our sexuality. All of this occurs in the context of our religious, cultural, and ethnic beliefs and practices. Many of us have strong feelings about what's right and wrong and what's acceptable or not acceptable about sexuality, sexual expression, and sexual activity. This, too, is influenced by our family of origin, our education as children, teens, and adults, and the experiences we've had as we have matured.

On the other hand, *sexual functioning* describes what we do as sexual beings. There is a whole language around this phrase. Most people have their own language for sexual functioning and use euphemisms to describe what they do. For example, many couples talk about their "intimate life," which comprises their "sexual activity" as well as the feelings of connectedness that flow from that. Or they may use that phrase because they're embarrassed to say the words "sexual activity" or "sexual intercourse." Many people refer to "making love," which may be, to them, a more acceptable way of saying that they engage in sexual activity. The phrase *sexual activity* is confusing in many ways; for some people it means having intercourse, while for others it may mean masturbation, alone or with a partner. For others, it may involve only oral sex without genital penetration.

The importance that we, as individuals and couples, place on sexual functioning tends to ebb and flow throughout our lives. At the beginning of a relationship, sex is often of high importance, and most of us can recall with fondness those first few months of a new relationship where every kiss, touch, and glance made our pulses race. But when raising a young family, many women find that sex takes a backseat to the myriad other roles and responsibilities they have. This can cause stress in a relationship when members of the couple have different levels of sexual desire. Menopause also presents changes to sexuality and sexual functioning at a time when a woman's partner may be experiencing his or her own changes. Acute or chronic illness poses another challenge, and some couples choose to ignore their sexual needs and desires in the face of health challenges for fear of causing damage or pain to their partners.

Cancer and Sexuality

Some people may think that these two words—sexuality and cancer—don't go together. This is probably because they haven't experienced cancer or because they have an image of sexuality as being related to the more sensationalized images we see in the media or to reproduction. If sexuality is the expression of ourselves as human beings, then it's important to consider that cancer and its treatments don't take away the experience of being a sexual person. Cancer may change the way we see ourselves as sexual beings but not necessarily in a negative way. Today, the success or failure of cancer treatment is not judged solely on the basis of cure but also on how it affects quality of life for patients, their partners, and their families. Cancer can have a profound effect on all aspects of quality of life, including physical, psychological, and social dimensions.

The physical location of the cancer can profoundly affect how a woman sees herself as a sexual being. Gynecologic cancer affects a woman's reproductive organs, which also are her sexual organs. Breast cancer affects a part of the body that represents femininity to many women, and alterations to the structure of the breast can profoundly affect her self-image and body image. Other cancers may seem less likely to affect sexual functioning, but because the heart, mind, and soul, as well as the body, play a part in sex, *any* cancer experience can affect how women perceive themselves and how they act out their sexuality and sexual feelings.

The Stages of Illness

As with all other illnesses, cancer has its own unique stages. Sexuality and sexual functioning are affected at every stage of the cancer journey. The time surrounding diagnosis is usually one of crisis. When multiple tests are being done to diagnose a particular cancer, a woman may find that she's under too much stress to enjoy sexual thoughts or sexual activity; yet, other women may find that sexual activity is a distraction and a way to connect with themselves and their partner in a pleasurable way and put aside fears and uncertainties. When the cancer diagnosis is made, life is forever changed, and a woman must learn a whole new way of being as she works with the healthcare team to develop a plan for care and treatment. For many, a diagnosis of cancer initially presents a very real threat to life, and thoughts of death are very real. Many women find that even thinking about sex seems contradictory. Others find solace and comfort in the arms of their partner. Touch and sensation may take on new meaning in the face of this threat to life.

Cancer treatments can have significant effects on sexual feelings and expression. The most common treatments for cancer—surgery, radiation, chemotherapy, and hormonal manipulation—all have the potential to affect how the body works. The impact may be temporary, long-lasting, or even permanent. Treatments can affect nerves, blood vessels, muscles, skin, bones, and hormone levels. The mind, too, can be affected, and the psychological and emotional impact of the treatments may persist for many months or even years. Some women put sex on the back burner and, over time, might not "revisit" themselves as sexual beings. Other women mourn the changes in their lives and try to stay connected to their partners and their own bodies through whatever means they can find, depending on their health and the severity of treatment side effects.

When treatment is over, the "chronic" phase of cancer begins. Many women find that over time, the body heals and returns to something resembling normalcy. But this can be a time of great uncertainty, when altered sensations can cause panic that the cancer is back. Some women do experience recurrence, and once again there is a crisis as expectations or hopes are crushed and a transition to quality versus length of life may need to be made.

But thanks to dramatic advances in cancer detection and treatment, more and more people are surviving cancer. According to the American Cancer Society (2008), at least 10.5 million Americans with a history of cancer were alive in 2003, and between 1996 and 2002, survival rates were up 51% over previous decades. There are many myths associated with cancer survival, including the myth that once treatment is over, a woman should go back to life as it was before and also should return to her precancer sense of self, including sexual functioning. The reality is that some women return to their previous levels of sexual functioning, and others don't. Some find that the alterations they needed to make during treatment or recovery from treatment have opened up a new world, and they incorporate these changes as permanent features of an expanded or different sex life. For some women, the cessation of sexual activity during acute treatment is never addressed, and they don't attempt to return to their previous activities. For some, this may be a relief—perhaps sex wasn't important or enjoyable to them, and the cancer was a welcome excuse to avoid it. Others don't know that there's help available to assist them in finding solutions to problems they encounter with treatment or recovery. Some women's healthcare providers never even ask patients if they have any questions or need help dealing with changes in their sexual functioning. If you've experienced sexual problems during or after cancer, you're not alone. Almost half of all cancer survivors report ongoing problems with sexual functioning; these problems are physical, emotional or psychological, and social.

What Can You Expect From This Book?

I'm a passionate believer that all people who experience cancer—patients and their partners—deserve to have their issues with sexual functioning addressed and resolved in the best way possible. Every day, I counsel patients and their partners experiencing these very problems. This book explains the changes that many women with cancer experience and offers practical advice on how to handle these changes. Each chapter describes the experience of a woman with a particular kind of cancer. But the experience isn't applicable only to women with that kind of cancer. Even if you've experienced a different kind of cancer, you'll find yourself relating to that woman's feelings and her experiences with a variety of problems, including loss of libido, physical pain during and after treatment, and struggles communicating with a partner. So make sure you read every chapter of this book even if you think it doesn't apply directly to you, because all chapters include information that applies to different types of cancer. And ask your partner to read it, too. Why is this important? Because there are some universal experiences for those who have cancer that are not different by type of cancer. For instance, fatigue is a universal response to many treatments, and body image is something that many women are very concerned about and is almost always affected by cancer.

This book has three parts. The first deals with sexual functioning and describes "how things work," so that you'll be able to better understand the terms commonly used in talking about sexuality and sexual functioning. The second part highlights the different feelings—physical and emotional—that women with cancer may experience. These include changes in body image, loss of sexual desire, alterations in arousal, changes in orgasmic response, pain, and the emotional responses to these changes. There's also a chapter on how to communicate with a potential partner about a sensitive and often emotionally laden topic. Issues facing lesbians with cancer are addressed, as well as the interaction between fertility and sexuality. The third part presents specific strategies for the woman with cancer, including drugs and other therapies used to treat sexual problems, communication strategies and exercises, and additional resources for where to find help. Because the partners of women with cancer experience their own individual issues, there's also a chapter in this section for the partner of the woman with cancer.

Today, most women who receive a cancer diagnosis will go on to survive, and in time, the memory of cancer and its treatments will fade. Sexuality is a part of life, and women deserve to continue to express themselves as sexual beings in loving relationships. This book gives you the information and tools you need to reclaim your sex life after the challenges of cancer.

Reference

American Cancer Society. (2008). *Cancer facts and figures, 2008.* Retrieved November 26, 2008, from http://www.cancer.org/docroot/STT/content/STT_1x_Cancer_Facts_and_Figures_2008.asp

CHAPTER 2

How Do Things Work?

To talk about sex, we need to know about the parts and processes involved in sexual activities. We know quite a bit about the parts: the female and male reproductive organs. And we know something about how they work, but even in this area, we are learning all the time. Do we know how diseases like cancer affect sexuality? Yes, in part, we do. But there is still lots to learn. So let's start at the beginning with the female (and for completeness) the male sexual organs.

Sexual Anatomy

Women have breasts, and below the waist are the pubic mound (or mons), the vulva (made up of the clitoris, the labia majora and minora [inner and outer lips], and the entrance to the vagina), and then internally the vagina and cervix. The cervix connects to the uterus and uterine (fallopian) tubes. The ovaries lie in the abdomen and produce the hormones that influence sexual functioning.

The breasts grow and develop during the years of puberty. They are described as secondary sex characteristics. The breasts are mostly fat and a special tissue called mammary glands. The mammary glands produce milk after a baby is born, and the fat gives breasts their size and shape. Each breast has a nipple on it that is surrounded by a colored area of skin called the areola. The nipples and areolae have many nerve endings that are very sensitive and play a role in sexual arousal.

The genital organs in the woman have external and internal parts. On the outside is the pubic mound, or mons. It is a fatty pad that lies over the pubic bone and after puberty is covered with hair. Lying below the mons are two fleshy folds of skin (called the labia majora) that run backwards to the entrance to the vagina. These also usually are covered with hair. They lie over the inner lips (the labia minora). The inner lips surround the opening of the urethra (which carries urine from the bladder) and the entrance to the vagina. This area also has a lot of nerve endings and a rich blood supply. During sexual arousal, the whole area will swell and grow darker in color.

Where the inner labia meet in the front, just below the mons, is the clitoris. This organ has the highest number of nerves in the human body, even more than the number supplying the male penis. It used to be thought that the clitoris was a small organ, about the size of a pea. Many medical textbooks still show it that way. But we now know that the clitoris has a large part of itself hidden under the skin of the labia; in fact, there is clitoral tissue as far back as the entrance to the vagina on each side. Just a small part of the clitoris is visible on the outside, and it is partly covered by a hood.

The entrance to the vagina lies between the urethra in the front and the anus in the back. The vagina is a tube about three to five inches in length. The walls of the vagina are covered in mucosal tissue that also is richly supplied with blood, but this area does not contain many nerve endings. This is probably a good thing when you think about a 9-pound baby coming through the vagina! There are more nerves in the lower third of the vagina, near the entrance. In its normal resting state, the walls of the vagina touch each other. These walls have many folds, and the mucosal cells secrete a fluid to keep the vagina moist.

The cervix lies at the top of the vagina and serves as the entrance to the uterus. The cervix makes a fluid that lubricates the vagina. On either side of the cervix are two large groupings of nerves and blood vessels that supply the sexual organs. The uterus is a muscular organ, roughly the size and shape of a pear. The uterine tubes (also called the fallopian tubes) extend from each side of the uterus toward the ovaries. The ovaries produce eggs (ova) and sex hormones: estrogen, progesterone, and testosterone.

Let's briefly talk about the male sex organs. Externally are the penis and the scrotum. The scrotum contains the testicles, which produce the sex hormone testosterone. The penis consists of the shaft and the head (or glans), which may be covered by a foreskin. Some parents opt to have the foreskin removed when their sons are babies (referred to as circumcision). Running through the penis is the urethra, which carries urine and ejaculate to the outside. The internal organs are the vas deferens, which carries sperm to the prostate gland, the seminal vesicles, which make the fluid portion of the ejaculate; and the Cowper's glands, which produce a liquid during sexual arousal. An important internal organ is the prostate, which lies underneath the bladder and surrounds the urethra. The prostate makes fluid that forms part of the ejaculate and also aids in the process of expulsion of semen during ejaculation.

Hormonal Influences

The hypothalamus and pituitary gland in the brain control the secretion of hormones by the ovaries and testicles. These hormones (estrogens, progesterone, and testosterone) are important for various aspects of male and female sexuality and sexual functioning. Another hormone, prolactin, also is important for libido, and oxytocin is produced after orgasm. Women have higher levels of estrogen and progesterone than men but lower levels of testosterone.

Estrogen is involved in the maturation of sexual organs, the development of the breasts and body hair, and the regulation of the menstrual cycle. Estrogen also is called the hormone of arousal because it increases the secretion of lubrication in the vagina.

The Sexual Response Cycle

The brain often is described as the biggest sex organ, in part because of the role that the brain plays in sexual thoughts and fantasies, sexual desire, and the interpretation of sensations. Our modern understanding of human sexuality comes originally from the work of Masters and Johnson in the 1960s. They developed a model of human sexual functioning comprising four parts. These stages (excitement, plateau, orgasm, and resolution) were described as the same for men and women and were thought to occur in a linear fashion with one stage following the other. These stages essentially are made up of episodes of increased blood supply to sexual organs, as well as muscle contractions.

The Excitement Stage

In this first stage, the heart beats faster and blood pressure increases. Blood flows into the tissues of the sexual organs, causing swelling. The breasts increase in size, and the skin of the chest may flush. The tissues of the genitals all increase in size. The clitoris enlarges, the large outer lips flatten outward, and the inner lips swell. The upper two-thirds of the vagina grow bigger, and moisture seeps out of the walls of the vagina.

The Plateau Phase

This is a state of advanced arousal where breathing becomes rapid. The lower third of the vagina swells, making the entry to the vagina smaller. The upper two-thirds of the vagina continue to grow. The uterus moves into an upright position. The inner lips become darker from the increased blood flow. The clitoris withdraws under the clitoral hood. The breasts continue to grow bigger in size and the nipples flatten out.

Orgasm

This is a phase of muscular contractions and intense sensations. The pelvic muscles contract 15–20 times; the first contractions usually are strong and close together and are followed by three or more slower contractions. The muscles of the anal sphincter also contract, as does the uterus itself. Both breathing and heart rates peak, and the person feels intense pleasure radiate throughout the body.

The Resolution Phase

In this final phase, the body returns to its normal nonaroused state. Muscle tension disappears, and heart rate, blood pressure, and respiration return to normal. Blood moves out of the pelvic organs, and everything returns to its normal state and color.

Of note is that this model makes no mention of any cognitive or psychological component; the brain is missing. This is evident in that it does not include a stage of desire or libido. A student of Masters and Johnson, Helen Singer Kaplan, introduced the idea of *desire* to the human sexual response cycle. She suggests that there are three stages: desire, excitement, and orgasm. Singer states that the subjective feeling of desire is an important part of the sexual response. In this model, *excitement* represents increased blood flow to the genitals causing lubrication in women. *Orgasm* is a series of muscular contractions. Unlike Masters and Johnson, whose model is linear with one stage following another, Kaplan's model has three independent phases that do not follow one another. So, it is possible to experience excitement without first feeling desire, but most people interpret her model as being linear because it is presented in a linear fashion.

Rosemary Basson developed a more recent interpretation of the female sexual response cycle. This model is presented as a circle with much emphasis on women's thoughts and feelings (see Figure 1). Basson suggests that women have many reasons to be receptive sexually, including feelings of well-being, emotional intimacy, and lack of negative feelings from avoiding sex. This motivation allows a woman to be receptive to sexual advances from her partner. These advances are interpreted by the woman both physically and mentally, and arousal then occurs. It may be at this stage that the woman realizes she actually wants to be sexual, rather than desire (or libido) occurring first and leading to sexual activity. Basson suggests that orgasm is not necessary for sexual satisfaction for women, but satisfaction may come from seeing one's partner enjoying the experience. Satisfaction is suggested to increase motivation for future sexual encounters and makes the woman more willing the next time.

Conclusion

This chapter has described the anatomy and functioning of the sex organs. But sexuality is so much more than body parts and how they work. Sexuality in women is a complex phenomenon with anatomic, hormonal, and behavioral aspects. It's important to know how things work and where things are so that you understand what might happen if your body is altered by cancer or its treatments. Cancer not only affects the body parts discussed here but also alters the way we respond to sexual touch and feelings.

Figure 1. Basson's Sex Response Cycle, Showing Responsive Desire Experienced During the Sexual Experience as Well as Variable Initial (Spontaneous) Desire

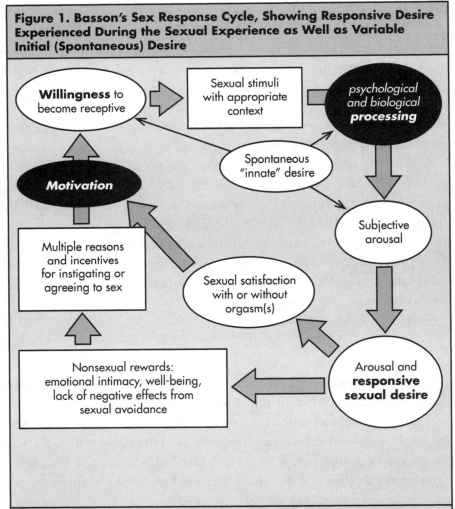

A woman's reasons for instigating or agreeing to sex include a desire to express love, to receive and share physical pleasure, to feel emotionally closer, to please the partner and to increase her own well-being. This leads to a willingness to find and consciously focus on sexual stimuli. These stimuli are processed in the mind, influenced by biological and psychological factors. The resulting state is one of subjective sexual arousal. Continued stimulation allows sexual excitement and pleasure to become more intense, triggering desire for sex itself: sexual desire, absent initially, is now present. Sexual satisfaction, with or without orgasm, results when the stimulation continues sufficiently long and the woman can stay focused, enjoys the sensation of sexual arousal and is free from any negative outcome such as pain.

Note. From "Women's Sexual Dysfunction: Revised and Expanded Definitions," by R. Basson, 2005, *Canadian Medical Association Journal, 172*(10), p. 1328. Copyright 2005 by Canadian Medical Association. Reprinted with permission.

PART TWO

What Happened? Cancer and Sex

In this section, you will meet 10 women and their partners. All these women have had cancer and have experienced some kind of sexual difficulty as a result of the cancer or its treatment.

You will have an intimate view of their lives and struggles, as well as explanations of why they are experiencing sexual problems and how they overcame them or adapted to them.

Dr. Katz's explanations are followed by tips that can help you as you try to deal with the same kinds of issues; Take-Away Points are included to provide real and useful information for sexual and treatment-related problems.

CHAPTER 3

Altered Body Image

When I look in the mirror, I see a changed person.

A significant part of the experience for women with breast cancer relates to how they feel about their bodies. Body image is a complicated thing. What we see in the mirror is not necessarily what's really there. What do I mean by this? Well, we all have images in our heads about how we look, and we often assign a value to this: too fat, too thin, too jiggly. We usually judge ourselves quite harshly.

We've been told so many things about what is beautiful and how we "should" look. Since we were children, we've heard messages from many different sources: our parents, grandparents, and siblings, friends, teachers, and coaches. The messages from the media are relentless: in particular, the media presents perfect images of women as the "ideal" even though these images have been touched up before going to print. The models and actresses we see as role models often are really young, have unhealthy lifestyles, and do not show us what we know to be "actual" women.

This chapter tells the story of Sheila, 55, who had a mastectomy for breast cancer followed by breast reconstruction. You'll learn from her story

- How to cope with changes to the body
- How to learn to accept this "new" body.

Sheila's Story

Shelia is 55 years old and works as a legal secretary in a large law firm. Two years ago, she married Paul; she'd been divorced for about 10 years before that and is still in the throes of what she calls "an extended honeymoon" with her second husband. Sheila has been having regular annual mammograms for a number of years. Her mother had breast cancer, and Sheila's been vigilant with her checkups. Six months ago, she felt something in her breast while in the shower. She immediately made an appointment with her family physician, who ordered a diagnostic mammogram, which showed something suspicious. A biopsy confirmed a diagnosis of breast cancer.

Sheila was devastated that, at this point in her life when she was so happy, something so bad was happening to her. She felt this enormous sense of urgency to "do something" and asked the surgeon to perform the surgery as soon as possible. Sheila withdrew into herself in the two weeks before her surgery. She'd told her boss, a partner in the law firm where she worked, and requested that he keep her diagnosis confidential. She planned to take six weeks off from work after the surgery and wanted as few people as possible to know about it.

Take-Away Points

- You don't have to tell everyone at the same time. And you don't have to tell anyone anything. Those close to you will quickly figure out that something's wrong, so perhaps you can tell one or two people and then they can tell your other friends.
- Telling people about your cancer can be really tiring and emotionally draining. That's why telling one or two friends or relatives and letting them get the word out can be a good thing.

Dr. Katz Explains

After a cancer diagnosis, it's quite common to want to do something right away. There are times when surgery is urgent or even an emergency. But often, there's time to allow for some reflection and to find out exactly what your options are, as well as what the consequences of the different types of surgery may be.

Some women want as few people as possible to know about their cancer. They try to keep it secret and only tell a few close friends and anyone who has to know, like an employer. This has both positive and negative consequences; on the one hand, keeping it quiet limits the number of people who'll ask how you are, and you won't have to talk about it a lot. On the other hand, keeping it quiet also limits the number of people who can offer support. But the choice is an individual one to make, and you can tell a lot of people or restrict this news to a very few.

The Surgery Draws Near

Paul was very supportive in the weeks leading up to the surgery. In many ways, he felt quite lost and wasn't sure what to do to help Sheila. She'd withdrawn from him, too, and he tried to be respectful of this; they'd only known each other for close to three years, and this was really the first major challenge they had to face. Paul's first wife was an alcoholic, and he'd learned to steer clear of her when the going got tough; he fell back into that old pattern in this crisis with Sheila.

One week before her surgery, Sheila had an appointment with the surgeon who was going to do the mastectomy. The surgeon asked Sheila if she'd given any thought to whether she wanted reconstruction, and Sheila replied, "Of course." The nurse at the surgeon's office already had made an appointment for her with a plastic surgeon; this appointment took place immediately after her meeting with the breast surgeon.

The plastic surgeon's offices were plush and inviting, but Sheila hardly noticed her surroundings. She'd gone alone to all her appointments, and this one was no different. Paul had wanted to go with her and support her, but she told him that he was too busy at work to take off time, and anyway, she was just fine. He backed off but felt really bad that she was doing all of this by herself. At the plastic surgeon's office, the receptionist warmly greeted Sheila, who was taken into a room within minutes of her arrival.

Dr. Katz Explains

Take-Away Point

Women sometimes try to do everything by themselves and keep their partner at arm's length. At a time like this, just before surgery, many women struggle to find a sense of control in their lives; choosing to make all decisions by themselves may be one way of taking control. But this shuts out one's partner, who is also feeling out of control and scared about what the future holds.

- If you don't want to take someone with you to the appointment, ask your healthcare provider if you can record your conversation with him/her. You can use a tape recorder for this. Many people find this helpful so they can go over what was said as many times as they need to make sense of it all.

Taking a partner or trusted friend to medical appointments serves some important functions: four ears often are better than two, and having someone else there to listen to the information from healthcare providers is very helpful. Your companion can then discuss with you what was said at the appointment. When you have so many questions, the words of the healthcare provider can get lost in the noise in your head; having someone there who is a little removed from the situation really can help. The person with you can take notes as a reminder for you afterward.

Choosing a Breast

The plastic surgeon didn't keep Sheila waiting very long, and soon they were talking about the details of reconstructive surgery. Sheila was presented with two options: a TRAM flap procedure where skin and fat are taken from the abdominal area and transferred to the side where her breast had been removed, or she could have a saline implant inserted to replace her breast. The surgeon outlined the pros and cons of each and suggested that because Sheila was quite thin and didn't have much fat on her belly, the implant would be a better choice. Sheila agreed immediately and was pleased to learn that the implant would be placed at the time of the mastectomy. This would mean that her surgery would take longer, but it also meant that she only had to have one operation. She signed the consent form and was almost out of the examination room when a nurse came in and asked if Sheila wanted to see photographs of other women who had the same procedure. Sheila refused; she was eager to get back to work and thought that this would be a waste of time. What could looking at pictures add? She just wanted this whole thing to be over.

Dr. Katz Explains

Many women want to have immediate reconstruction after a mastectomy. The thought of having everything done at once is somewhat comforting. Because she was thin, Sheila in effect didn't have a choice of procedure and so consented to the saline implant. The one mistake that Sheila made at this appointment was to refuse to look at photographs of other women who had this procedure. These can be very helpful in presenting a realistic picture of what happens when one has a saline implant. Without this reality check, many women either have unrealistic expectations of what a reconstructed breast looks like or have no real picture of it in their minds. This can lead to disappointment later, as we shall see with Sheila. Pretending that something's not happening or not paying enough attention can lead to problems accepting and adapting later on.

Take-Away Points

- Ask to see photos of other women who've had the same procedure or surgery as you're having. And don't just look at the breasts; in the TRAM flap procedure, there will be scars on the lower abdomen, too.
- Check out a local support group for women with breast cancer. There will be women in the group who'll tell you what their experience was like and how they feel about their breasts and body now.
- Even though you may think that avoiding some of the issues related to treatment decisions (such as looking at pictures of other women who've had this surgery) is helpful, we know that being active and engaged in your choices ultimately makes for a better recovery.

The Surgery

Soon the day of Sheila's surgery arrived. Paul drove her to the hospital, and she was very quiet in the car. This wasn't unexpected; she had been really uncommunicative since she was diagnosed. She insisted that Paul not wait around, but he came in with her and stayed until they took her to the operating room. He then went to work, where, for the most part, he stared at his computer screen and waited for the call that she was out of surgery.

Sheila woke up after the surgery in a fog of pain and confusion. After a few minutes, she remembered where she was and why, but the pain persisted. The nurse in the recovery room explained about the morphine pump that she could use to increase her pain medication, and soon she was dozing through the pain. Her chest felt as if it was being crushed by a band of heat, and every now and then her hand touched the thick bandages that went from just under her arms almost to her stomach. Soon Paul was there, and she smiled weakly as he took her hand.

Sheila was discharged within a few days and asked for help from the visiting nurse program; she wanted assistance when changing the dressing and didn't want to ask Paul to do it. Her recovery was slower than she expected, and she found that she needed to nap most afternoons. Paul felt that there was not much for him to do; he had taken off two weeks of work to help Sheila, but all he found himself doing was making dinner every night. She still didn't talk much about how she was feeling or what she was thinking. Paul waited it out; he was confident that the old Sheila would return and things would go back to normal.

Dr. Katz Explains

Many women expect too much of themselves and are surprised when they don't bounce back immediately after the surgery. Surgery and the anesthesia in particular take a lot out of you, and you really do need to take all the time you need to recover.

Many women don't want their partner to see the surgical site and need help to change the dressing or clean the area. There is no right or wrong way to handle this, and professional help is available for such things. But keeping your partner removed from what is happening to you physically can also increase the distance between you emotionally. Some partners don't want to see the scar or anything else; it may even make them squeamish. But other partners would be quite happy to be involved and may want to help with dressing changes or anything else that is asked of them.

And What Comes Next . . .

Sheila gets a call from her surgeon, who tells her that based on the results of the pathology tests done on her breast tissue, she has to get chemotherapy. She knew this was a possibility, but she's still upset now that she knows for certain. Her recovery continues. She no longer has a dressing over her reconstructed breast and is going for daily physical therapy to help with mobility of the arm on that side. She's concerned about the amount of swelling in the reconstructed breast, but the plastic surgeon tells her this is normal and she'll continue to see improvements over the coming weeks and months.

She starts her chemotherapy exactly six weeks after her surgery. Her physical recovery has gone well, and she's feeling almost back to normal. She's extended her sick leave from work, and her boss there has been very understanding. Her relationship with Paul, however, isn't what it once was. She remains distant, and they're both struggling with how to reestablish the closeness they once had. Sheila finds it difficult to open up to him about her feelings. He doesn't know what to do to reach her even though he's tried everything he can think of. Romantic dinners at restaurants don't seem to have worked; she's concerned about their financial situation and thinks it's a waste of money. He tried buying her flowers, but she made a cutting comment about flowers and funerals so he hasn't tried that again.

Dr. Katz Explains

Depending on the nature of the cancer found in the breast and the tissue that was removed, some women have to undergo chemotherapy. These treatments usually begin after about six weeks when the physical healing has taken place. The emotional healing is another story.

This couple seems to be drifting apart and not talking to each other. He tries one thing, and she rebuffs him. She's done most of this by herself, which was her choice, but he feels left out. His ex-wife was an alcoholic, and their communication patterns weren't constructive. He's fallen into the same sort of pattern in this relationship with Sheila. She withholds and he tries to reach her and she rebuffs him; he tries something else, and once again she pushes back.

Take-Away Points

- At times of crisis, it's easy to fall into old patterns of behavior and communication. And at times like this, you probably don't have the energy to get into long discussions about feelings and the past.
- But if you're not talking to the person closest to you, then something's wrong. Your partner may not understand exactly what you're going through, but he does want to help and support you.
- Cutting out your partner makes him feel that you're punishing him for something he hasn't done.

The "S" Word

Paul misses the closeness that they once had, as well as the sex. There's been no sex since she was diagnosed almost nine weeks ago. He's reluctant to bring up the topic but misses her body and sex so much. The other thing that's really bothering him is that she no longer undresses in front of him. When she prepares for bed, she goes into the bathroom and closes the door firmly behind her. In the morning, she dresses in the walk-in closet.

Dr. Katz Explains

Even though his wife has gone through a lot with the diagnosis and surgery and now chemotherapy, Paul still wants and needs her sexually. This is not abnormal or insensitive; their relationship is fairly new, and sex is a way of expressing love for a partner. It's also a way to release tension and relax, and it makes us feel good and connected to the one we love.

Sheila has stopped undressing in front of Paul. This seemingly small act has large effects. Being naked in front of our partner is a sharing of something precious and special. Most of us don't show our naked body freely to anyone other than our partner or perhaps some very close friends. Our partners also find the sight of our naked bodies to be visually stimulating, despite the jiggles and wrinkles that time has added. In the case of Sheila and Paul, because he's not seen her naked since her surgery and hasn't seen her reconstructed breast, he may not have a realistic image in his mind of what it looks like. He may imagine something that isn't there at all, and this can potentially alter his reaction when and if he eventually is allowed to see her new breast.

Hair Today and Gone Tomorrow

Sheila starts chemotherapy. She's prepared for nausea but doesn't have any, probably because of a cocktail of drugs she takes before and after her treatments. She waits nervously for her hair to fall out, and that starts almost two weeks to the day after starting chemotherapy. The first clumps of hair lie on the shower floor early on a Tuesday morning. Sheila's shocked at how this affects her; she stands for a few minutes with the hot water flowing over her back and sobs, grateful that the water covers the sounds of her distress. She tells Paul later that day that she needs him to shave her head; she doesn't want to go through this one day at a time.

That evening Paul uses a hair clipper to shave her head. He's glad that he's standing behind her as he does this; he's not sure that he wants her to see his face. But he's so glad to have this opportunity to touch her, something that he's not been able to do for almost three months now. As the clipper does its job, his hands move over her head, and in this task that is centered on something painful, he feels joy as he touches her. He tells her how much he has missed her and their life before the breast cancer. He cries as he describes how lonely he has felt. Sheila admits that she, too, has been lonely and how difficult it has been for her to reach out and ask for support.

Dr. Katz Explains

At last Sheila has asked for help. In asking Paul to shave her head, she has actually given him a huge gift. For the first time in many months, he's able to touch her in an intimate way, and it brings him to tears. Sheila allows herself to open up just a little and tells him that she has found it hard to ask for help. It is interesting how out of something really painful for a woman—the loss of hair—come the first glimmerings of touch and understanding.

Hair Where?

A week later, Sheila notices that her pubic hair is starting to fall out. She's completely unprepared for this and is once again brought to tears. She mentions this to one of the nurses when she has her next treatment and is shocked when the nurse tells her this is completely normal. Why did no one warn her about this? It's as if a dam has broken, and Sheila starts to cry. She tells the nurse that she's really struggling with all the changes that she sees in her body. She feels let down because what she thought would happen has not. She hates her reconstructed breast and regrets that she even had that as part of her surgery. The nurse sits and listens, and when Sheila finally stops talking, she gently suggests that she should see one of the counselors that work at the cancer center. To the nurse's surprise, Sheila agrees to this and schedules an appointment for the following week when she does not have chemotherapy.

Take-Away Points

- Your healthcare provider may be waiting for you to ask the questions; you may have to make the first move.
- A simple statement like "I have some questions about XXXX (sex, pubic hair, etc.)" will open the door.

Dr. Katz Explains

Most women who have chemotherapy are completely unprepared for the loss of pubic hair. They expect the hair on their head to fall out, and many are proactive as Sheila was and actually shave it off instead of witnessing the slow loss in chunks and wisps. But pubic hair too?

The loss of pubic hair for many women is a violation of their adult selves. Now, it's true that many women shave or wax part or all of their pubic hair, but doing this by choice is a far cry from losing it as part of treatment. It also presents some unique challenges to how women see themselves as sexual beings. Without pubic hair, many women see themselves as little girls, and little girls aren't sexual. So for many women, bare genitals present a real challenge to sexual contact with their partners. This may seem to defy logic: even without pubic hair, you are still a woman by virtue of your age and experience. But feelings, especially feelings about oneself, aren't logical.

It's not clear why nurses and other healthcare providers don't warn all women that this loss of pubic hair is possible. They all tell women that the hair on the head will fall out. Healthcare providers are people, too, and they come to the work they do with values, attitudes, and beliefs that are, at times, conservative or shameful. Believe it or not, your nurse, oncologist, or radiation therapist may be too embarrassed to talk about sex or body parts. It may be really difficult for them because you're older than they are, and they feel that asking about it would be disrespectful. They may worry that you'll think that they are being rude if they ask a question about your sex life. Or they may just not have the words or the confidence to have an open discussion about it. Most likely they're waiting for *you* to bring up the subject, and then they'll take their lead from you. If you don't ask and they don't ask, the result is deafening silence.

Dr. Katz Explains

The breast with the implant will look and feel different. For a start, it'll be firmer and perkier than the normal breast of a 55-year-old woman. The reconstructed breast also is not likely to have a nipple, as this is usually tattooed or surgically applied with transplanted tissue sometime after the surgery. The reconstructed breast also will have a scar from the surgery, and the sensation when that breast is touched will be altered. Sheila may have areas where the skin is numb with no feeling or feels quite rubbery. There may be sensitive areas where every now and then it feels like electricity is going through the skin.

Now, Sheila may have been warned about this, but it's well known that at times of crisis, like just before surgery, we hear very little of what we're told. Remember my advice to bring along that second pair of ears? That might have served Sheila well. But this time when the nurse suggests that Sheila may benefit from counseling, Sheila hears and agrees to see someone.

Counseling Alone

Sheila doesn't tell Paul she's going to the counseling appointment. Things have been better between them since he shaved her head, and she's able to open up a little to him at night before they go to sleep. She's still not comfortable undressing in front of him, and since she now has no pubic hair, she's even more careful to lock the bathroom door. The counselor seems a bit surprised when Sheila arrives at the appointment by herself. Sheila talks hesitantly about her feelings since the diagnosis. The counselor asks probing questions, and soon Sheila finds herself talking openly about how disappointed she is with her reconstructed breast. She also talks about the shock she felt when her pubic hair fell out. She's surprised to find herself being so open about something so private, but it feels good to express her feelings. At the end of the session, she agrees to bring Paul with her to her next appointment.

Dr. Katz Explains

Once again Sheila keeps things to herself. By not telling Paul that she's going for counseling, she's excluding him. The counselor seemed to have expected her to come with her husband and asked that she bring him with her the next time. Most counselors will want to see the patient and her partner; this is a couple's issue. But having one or more sessions alone with the patient and one or two sessions with just the partner is often a good way to move the counseling along in a constructive way.

It's Sometimes About the Partner

Paul's a little hurt when Sheila tells him that she has seen the counselor and that she wants him to go to her next appointment. He is feeling really left out of her life and this experience, but he's pleased that she wants him to be there next time. He's willing to do anything to get her back; his loneliness is causing him such pain, and he feels guilty thinking about his needs given what she is going through.

Take-Away Points

- Remember that your partner is going through this, too—obviously not in the same way that you are, but it's really hard to see someone that you love in physical or emotional pain.
- When a couple's not sharing thoughts and feelings, there's lots of room for misunderstandings and confusion.

Dr. Katz Explains

It's often very difficult for the partner to say or do the right thing. There are plenty of opportunities for guilt, and Paul is feeling just that. He misses her and what their life was before the cancer. But she's the one who has gone through the physical and emotional pain and trauma.

Understanding Is Everything

The session with the counselor goes better than Paul ever expected. With gentle probing questions, the counselor encourages Sheila to talk to Paul about her feelings and fears. Paul's surprised to hear that she's so unhappy with her "new" breast. He has not even seen it and assumed that her distance was because of what she was going through with chemotherapy. He also thought that she was okay with her hair loss and is stunned when she tells him with difficulty that her pubic hair also is gone. For a moment he almost laughs but stops himself and feels the tears come to his eyes. He reaches out to her and pulls her into his arms. For an instant he feels her body stiffen in protest, but then she lets go and allows him to hold her for the first time in months.

Dr. Katz Explains

Because Sheila kept her feelings to herself, Paul really had little understanding of what she was going through. He did not know how bad she was feeling or how traumatized she has been by the changes in her body.

When two people do not communicate, there is ample opportunity for misperceptions and wrong assumptions. Paul thought that Sheila was struggling with the chemotherapy when she actually was struggling with her body image, which was negative. He assumed that because she had shaved her head, she was okay with the hair loss. How could he know that she was so distressed by the loss of her pubic hair? He had not seen that or even known that it was possible or had happened.

These two people, both struggling and lonely in their solitude, finally find each other in the counselor's office. Probably it was not soon enough, but certainly it was not too late. Their journey will continue, and, with some help, hopefully they will find each other again.

CHAPTER 4

Loss of Sexual Desire

Sex is the last thing on my mind right now.

It's common to experience changes in sexual desire, or libido, when you're confronted with any type of stress, including illness. Many women experience a loss of sexual desire both during and after cancer treatment, and they're often surprised that, even when they feel better, this aspect of their lives doesn't automatically return to what it was before they were diagnosed with cancer. Loss of libido is the most common complaint I hear from women who seek help. They just don't feel like having sex, they don't think about sex—for many, it's simply the last thing on their minds.

Libido is a complex phenomenon; it's both a physical and mental "feeling," and many women find it difficult to describe. But when it's lacking, they often miss it, or their spouses or partners comment that they feel neglected because their partner never initiates sex or is unwilling to respond to sexual advances.

This chapter tells the story of Beatrice, who experiences loss of libido after treatment for colon cancer. In this chapter, you'll learn about

- The different factors that contribute to loss of libido
- What treatment options are available
- How to communicate with your partner about this issue.

Beatrice's Story

Beatrice is 48 years old and has been married to Mark, 51, for 25 years. They live in a large home on two acres of land about an hour outside a large midwestern city. Beatrice is a receptionist for a family physician in a nearby town. Mark works in the information technology department at a hospital in the city. They have one son, Jason, who is away at college.

Two years ago, Beatrice noticed some blood on the toilet tissue. Her periods had been irregular for some months, and she thought that the bleeding was related to menopause. When she mentioned this to the physician she worked for, he encouraged her to see a specialist. Within a month, she was diagnosed with colon cancer and had surgery to remove a medium-sized tumor in her ascending colon. She was left with a colostomy, a surgically created opening on the skin of her abdomen through which feces is excreted into a bag; initially she hoped that the bag would be temporary, but the extent of the surgery required that it be permanent. She also underwent six months of chemotherapy, and her doctors have told her that, while she is now cancer free, she'll need to be followed closely.

Beatrice struggles with living with an ostomy bag. She has had to change her style of dressing and must wear loose-fitting clothes to hide the bag, which fills up at times with gas or stool. She no longer dresses or undresses in front of Mark and spends a lot of time in the bathroom dealing with the bag at various points during the day.

Take-Away Points

- Working with stoma therapists is important, as they have the tools and knowledge to help you to avoid or fix problems.
- There are always new devices and improvements that stoma therapists can pass on to their clients.

Dr. Katz Explains

Depending on where the cancer was in the colon, the amount and consistency of the stool will differ. Learning to manage this is an important part of life after colon cancer surgery. People with ostomies learn which foods are more likely to produce gas or odors, how often to change their bags, and how to anticipate problems while at work or at social events.

Life Doesn't Feel "Normal"

Beatrice returned to work three months after completing her chemotherapy and initially worked part-time, but for the past year has been back to working full-time. She's frustrated that her energy level still isn't what it used to be before her diagnosis. Most days it's all she can do to come home from work, prepare dinner, and then sit in front of the television before going to bed at 10 pm.

Dr. Katz Explains

Fatigue—both physical and mental—is a common and long-lasting effect of surgery. Many people go back to work soon after treatment is over and expect to feel better and "back to normal" right away. But recovery can be a long process, and it might take many months or even longer before you start to feel better.

Take-Away Points

- Try to negotiate a graduated back-to-work schedule with your employer. If you have to resume your previous schedule earlier than you'd like, be forgiving of yourself when you get home. Try to have a short nap before tackling housework or making dinner. Realize that you're not going to be able to do everything you did before. You have experienced a significant challenge and must cut yourself some slack.
- Know that your body will tell you when you're overdoing things, and try to accept that there are going to be times when you can't keep the house as clean as you'd like or you won't be able to meet social obligations. Enlist the help of friends or relatives whenever possible. When people ask what they can do, ask them to help with a task, such as emptying the dishwasher, folding the laundry, or picking the kids up from school. Practical activities like this are much more helpful than receiving another bouquet of flowers or box of chocolates, and people like to feel useful.

Feeling Blue

Mark was wonderful when Beatrice was recovering from surgery and having chemotherapy. He took time off work to be with her and tried to go to all her chemotherapy appointments. He accompanied her to all her follow-up appointments and has been unfailingly upbeat about her chances of beating this. Beatrice is less optimistic about long-term survival; she tends to be more negative than Mark in many ways and is inclined to see the glass as half empty.

While she was undergoing chemotherapy, Beatrice had two sessions with a psychologist at the hospital. At the urging of her nurses, who thought she was depressed, Beatrice agreed to the counseling because it was simply easier than trying to deny that she needed it. The psychologist explained that Beatrice was experiencing a typical reaction to her diagnosis and suggested to Beatrice that, if her mood didn't improve, she might benefit from an antidepressant, which her family physician could prescribe. But Beatrice has never discussed this with her family physician, who tends to leave any cancer-related issues to the oncologist.

Dr. Katz Explains

Some people have a more negative outlook on life than others. They tend to see the worst in any situation. This negative outlook may mask depression. Depression is quite common after a cancer diagnosis and treatment, yet many people are ashamed to acknowledge that they're feeling depressed. Although medication may be the answer for some people, there are additional ways to cope with feelings of depression after a cancer diagnosis. For example, exercise can be very effective in reducing depression, as can talk therapy with a mental health professional.

Take-Away Points

- Fatigue can look and feel like depression, and depression can make you feel tired. It's important to figure out if you're tired or depressed—or both. Certain signs of depression are different from those of fatigue. For example, with depression, eating habits may change; you may eat significantly more or less than usual. Early waking also may be a sign of depression. Your primary care physician can help you to distinguish between fatigue and depression.
- Even if you tend to see the glass as half empty, you don't have to suffer with depression. Help is available.
- Dealing with depression can make a significant difference in recovery. Medications, such as antidepressants, and talking to a trained professional, such as a psychologist or social worker/counselor, can help.

He Wants It; She Doesn't

All of the things Beatrice has experienced as a result of her cancer, including her fatigue, depression, and embarrassment about her colostomy, have led to a significant loss of sexual desire. And this is the one issue where there is friction between Mark and Beatrice. Mark always has had a higher sex drive than Beatrice. There have been times over the course of their marriage when they could laugh about this, but there also have been times when this caused unhappiness. Once or twice it has been so bad that Mark insisted that Beatrice seek help. With this ultimatum, Beatrice would try to be more interested, and for a couple of months, things would improve from Mark's perspective. But then they would eventually slide back into their previous pattern.

Since Beatrice's surgery, their sex life has been nonexistent. At first, Mark accepted this. When he saw how sick Beatrice was during her chemotherapy, he figured sex obviously was out of the question. But now that it's been two years since her diagnosis, he wonders when things will get back to normal.

Dr. Katz Explains

It's not uncommon for each member of a couple to have differing levels of interest in sex. Many couples find a way of dealing with this by accommodating each others' needs to the best of their ability. But compromising and not really addressing the issue properly can lead to what experts call a "sex-starved" marriage, in which resentment and anger build and permeate other aspects of the relationship. Often the partner with the higher sex drive feels rejected and neglected and may shut down emotionally. The one with low sex drive often finds it hard to empathize with his or her partner and may think that the partner is being over demanding, hurtful, and disrespectful of the other's feelings.

When one partner experiences cancer, the sympathy and understanding that the well partner gives during the illness feels good, but these couples typically don't have meaningful discussions about what they're feeling with regard to their sex life; much is left unsaid, and misunderstanding builds.

Take-Away Points

- Even when only one partner experiences loss of libido, the problem is a couple's problem and can be solved only as a couple.
- After an argument or ultimatum, things may seem to improve, but changes usually are temporary, and the problem will continue.
- One partner's apparent acceptance of a period of little or no sexual activity may be comforting to the partner experiencing loss of libido, but this acceptance doesn't last forever, and ultimately, both partners will have unexpressed expectations that lead to more misunderstandings.

Things Reach a Head

Beatrice tries to avoid thinking about her lack of sexual desire. She knows that Mark is frustrated, but she still is surprised to one day discover him viewing pornography on the Internet. She's not sure if he knows that she saw him, but she finds this disgusting and is very upset. One night she angrily confronts him. Mark is stunned by her outburst. For the first time in many months, they sit down and talk about what's happening. Mark tries very hard to hold in his frustration; Beatrice has a hard time not crying. Mark tells her that he loves her very much, but he doesn't understand why she isn't interested in sex. While he has no intention of looking outside the marriage for sex, he has resorted to looking at pornography and masturbating as a way to release his sexual tension. Beatrice only says that she's tired all the time and just not interested in sex. He suggests that she speak to someone, and she agrees to make an appointment with her gynecologist.

Take-Away Points

- It's always better to have a sensitive discussion such as this before reaching a crisis.
- Couples should talk about sex outside the bedroom, using all the strategies discussed in Chapter 12.
- Talking to an objective outsider is often easier than talking to your partner.

Dr. Katz Explains

Attitudes toward pornography and masturbation within a relationship vary. The important thing here is that Mark has reached a breaking point and may even have wanted to be "caught" by Beatrice as a way of forcing a discussion.

Can Medication Help to Boost Desire?

Beatrice sees her gynecologist three weeks later. At the appointment, she is very tearful and says that she thinks Mark is going to leave her unless she regains interest in sex. She asks for medication that will increase her sex drive and explains that she read something in a women's magazine about a patch that increases sexual desire. The gynecologist examines her and finds nothing physically wrong. Her periods still are irregular but her vaginal tissues are pink and moist. The gynecologist explains that after all she's been through it's not surprising that she has little or no interest in sex. She tells Beatrice that no medication has been shown to be effective for lack of sexual desire, but there are some strategies that may be helpful. One of these is for Beatrice and Mark to do some reading on the topic, and she hands her a list of books. Beatrice seems doubtful that this is going to help; she had wanted a more immediate and tangible solution, but she agrees to do some reading and makes another appointment for two weeks later.

Dr. Katz Explains

It's natural to want to take medicine to fix the problem. But currently, no medication has been shown to be effective for increasing libido in women who still have their ovaries (note: this may change as clinical trials provide additional evidence). There is some evidence that women who have had their ovaries surgically removed can benefit from treatment with testosterone, one of the hormones produced by the ovaries. However, the trials that were done were small and lasted only a few weeks; women need to stay on the medication for an extended period of time, and the treatment can produce side effects, including enlargement of the clitoris, deepening of the voice, and increased risk of heart disease.

Beatrice still is menstruating and, therefore, is producing her own hormones that influence sexual desire (for more information on how hormones affect sexual function, see Chapter 1).

The bottom line is that libido or sexual desire is a complex phenomenon that involves the brain, the emotions we feel, and previous experiences. Solving the problem of low libido is complicated and not easily solved by a pill or potion.

Take-Away Points

- This is not a new problem for this couple; it's a continuation of previous behavior and feelings.
- Seemingly easy solutions like taking a pill or using a patch will not affect memories, stored feelings, or attitudes that have been there for years. Differences in sexual desire between partners can take time and much effort and energy to resolve.

An "Ah-Ha" Moment

One of the books Beatrice reads talks about how even if you don't feel like having sex, sometimes when you get going, it feels good and you enjoy it. This makes sense to Beatrice, and she finds herself reading quickly through the rest of the book. The book has suggestions for both the person with low desire as well as the person with high desire. Mark is a little more skeptical; he thinks that it's all in Beatrice's head, and if she just tried harder, she would be interested.

Take-Away Points

- This model is not intended to force women into being sexual with a partner for whom they don't care or at a time that's not appropriate.
- Good communication is an essential component of any sexual encounter; the woman must be able to tell her partner when something feels good, and her partner must listen if she asks for the contact to stop.
- Small steps, such as touching and kissing, can lead to increased sexual desire later.

Dr. Katz Explains

Many people think that to have any kind of sexual activity, you first have to "be in the mood." Many researchers have described desire or libido as the first stage of the "sexual response cycle." The work of Masters and Johnson was described in Chapter 1; they didn't even consider desire as part of their model. Helen Singer Kaplan included desire as the first stage of her three-part model. Both of these models are linear, meaning that one stage follows the next: there is a beginning stage and the other stages follow in order. But sexuality researchers' and therapists' understanding of this has changed in recent years.

In recent years, an interesting alternative "model" of female sexual response has been described (refer back to Figure 1). This diagram represents a cycle that begins with the woman being willing to be receptive to her partner. If this is so, and sexual stimuli (such as touching or kissing) occur at an appropriate time and place, the woman will think about it and perhaps start to feel some physical sensations that are pleasurable. It may be here that she starts to feel desire (not at the beginning). The diagram shows that sexual satisfaction for the woman, as well as nonsexual rewards that flow from the partner being satisfied and greater intimacy, result in motivation for the woman to do it again, which translates into future willingness to allow sexual touching.

This model has been well-received by sex therapists and their clients. It seems to make intuitive sense to many women who've noticed that often when they don't feel like having sex, allowing some touching does increase their desire, which, in turn, makes them more receptive at another time.

Getting Started on the Path Back to Sex

Beatrice returns to the gynecologist two weeks later. Things have not improved. What she read makes sense, but she isn't sure how to approach Mark sexually after all this time. She admits to the physician that she hasn't even been naked in front of Mark since before the surgery and is ashamed of her body with its new scars and the ostomy bag. The gynecologist suggests that Beatrice meet with the stoma therapist at the hospital where she had her surgery. Beatrice has spoken to the therapist on the phone, mostly to ask questions about supplies. She calls the therapist and makes an appointment for later in the week.

The stoma therapist, Dawn, quickly puts Beatrice at ease and soon they're talking very openly about a topic that Beatrice isn't comfortable with. Dawn acknowledges that Beatrice's feelings are common. Many people with an ostomy bag are concerned about their partner's response to the bag and are fearful of leakage and odor. These feelings interfere with feeling like a sexual being. Dawn has more reading material for Beatrice and also suggests a Web site (see Resources section in Chapter 16) where she can get additional information. Beatrice feels much better after this appointment. She also is somewhat embarrassed that she ignored this resource for so long. She shares the information with Mark, and he talks about his feelings about her ostomy for the first time.

Dr. Katz Explains

It's common to avoid being naked in front of your spouse or partner when you feel ashamed of your body. As discussed in Chapter 3, body image plays a role in sexual difficulties in many different cancers. One of the results of always concealing your body is that your partner is denied a visual source of pleasure. This can cause or magnify distancing in the relationship.

Beatrice and Mark have never really talked about her stoma and bag. Mark hasn't wanted to raise the topic for fear of causing her emotional pain, and the silence has gotten deeper over the years.

Take-Away Points

- Expert help usually is available, and these people are experts for a reason: They know a lot about a particular disease or condition and have seen others struggle with similar issues.
- Asking for help is not a sign of weakness.
- Fears about leakage and odor are common, and there are many ways to deal with this. Speaking to a stoma therapist will provide strategies that the patient often has not considered.
- Most of us have bodies that are different from what they were when we were young, and yet we still find our partners attractive. Somehow we don't grace our partners with the same emotions, and we think that they are judging us.
- Allowing your partner to talk about his or her feelings about scars and other issues can be very freeing because what you think your partner is feeling may not be accurate.

A New Nightgown and a Little Laughter

Take-Away Point

- Humor is so important in life and is especially helpful when dealing with a sensitive topic. Just be careful that the humor is shared and not directed only at one person.

That night at bedtime, Mark looks hopeful. Beatrice spends a long time in the bathroom before appearing in a new nightgown—one that's very different from the ankle-length flannel one she usually wears. She is tense, and Mark tries to make a joke about this being very different from their first time, when they could hardly wait to tear each other's clothes off. This helps to break the ice, and they laugh at the memory of long ago when they could hardly wait to have sex and Mark had dropped the condom onto the carpet and it was their only one and there were probably carpet fibers on the outside.

Dr. Katz Explains

There are many different ways to hide or camouflage an ostomy bag. Depending on what type of stool collects in the bag, some people are able to irrigate the stoma and then cap it; after doing this, they may not need to wear a bag for a period of time. This may require some modifications to intake of food and fluid.

Wearing a cummerbund or scarf tied around the torso also can hide the bag.

Using an opaque fabric cover over the ostomy bag also can hide the contents and feels softer than plastic.

Some people prefer to remain partially clothed during sexual activity; this can be achieved by wearing lingerie or a nightgown that is different from what you usually wear. For example, crotchless panties allow the vulva to be free while the area of the stoma is protected by the fabric.

Trying alternative positions for intercourse also may help. The woman-on-top position prevents pressure being applied to the stoma. The side-lying position (on the side of the stoma) allows the pouch to fall toward the surface and not come between the partners. The rear-entry position, either kneeling or lying, where the woman lays in front of her partner, also prevents placing pressure on the stoma or bag.

Some preparation may be necessary to clean the area around the stoma, empty and deodorize the bag, and ensure that it is securely fastened.

Over the next few months, things improved for Beatrice and Mark. She still has to make a conscious effort to think about and prepare for sex. Because she's often very tired by the end of the day, she and Mark have found that taking time for each other on a weekend afternoon has reduced the pressure on Beatrice. Mark's also learned to be more playful and finds that if he makes jokes, sometimes at his own expense, Beatrice is less serious about it and seems more receptive. There is hope.

CHAPTER 5

Arousal Disorders

It's as if I'm dead from the waist down.

Arousal is a vital part of a fulfilling sex life. It involves various physical processes, including blood flowing into the sexual organs, as well as hormonal and nervous system responses. Arousal may produce a pleasurable sensation of fullness and tingling and may be accompanied by swelling and engorgement in the sexual organs. In men, the most noticeable signal of arousal is an erection, whereas in women it is vaginal lubrication.

But arousal is about much more than just these most noticeable manifestations. Arousal is tied to several physical, psychological, and emotional factors. As illustrated in the following case, problems with arousal can have significant consequences for both individuals and couples. The good news is that arousal disorders can be successfully dealt with, and couples can return to a complete and fulfilling sex life.

This chapter tells the story of Mona, a 47-year-old woman who experiences problems with arousal and intimacy after being treated for cervical cancer. In this chapter, you'll learn

- How cancer treatments, including surgery and radiation, can affect the sexual organs as well as feelings of intimacy and arousal
- What questions to ask your healthcare providers about the effects your diagnosis and treatment might have on your sexual functioning
- How to communicate with your partner about what you're both feeling and experiencing surrounding your cancer and your sex life
- Specific exercises you can do to reestablish arousal, intimacy, and sexual pleasure.

Mona's Story

Mona, 47, is married to James, who is 48. They have 18-year-old twins, Jesse and Jill, and live in a well-kept suburban home in a large metropolitan city. The twins attend a local high school and are active in sports and other extracurricular activities. They plan to attend a nearby state college after high school graduation. Mona went back to work when the twins started school and enjoys her career as an administrative assistant in a large pharmaceutical company. After working for a large office-supply company for many years, James left this job to buy and run a discount retail store. He works long hours and has only a small staff to help him.

Mona started experiencing symptoms of menopause in her early 40s, but it was a relatively easy transition for her. She wasn't sad to see her period go, and she thankfully didn't experience the severe hot flashes and insomnia that her female coworkers complained about.

It's now 15 months after her last period and she's seen her physician for her annual check-up. She was somewhat surprised when her physician called her within a week and asked her to come in the following day to discuss the results of her tests. She has some abnormal cells on her cervix and needs to have further tests.

A week later, she sees a gynecologist and undergoes a colposcopy, which is a biopsy of the cervix. Over the next few days, she is very quiet. James tries to comfort her as best he can, but she seems withdrawn, like she's avoiding his attempts at conversation. After 20 years of marriage, he knows that pushing her will only make her more withdrawn, so he decides to wait this out. He does insist on accompanying her to her follow-up appointment with the uro-gynecologist the following week.

The news they receive isn't good. Mona has invasive cervical cancer and will require a radical hysterectomy followed by radiation therapy about six weeks later. Both James and Mona are in shock, and when asked if they have any questions, they shake their heads and are ushered out of the office and told that they'll be contacted about a surgery date. They go home, where James breaks down, and Mona finds herself comforting him and assuring him that things will be all right.

Dr. Katz Explains

Each of us has a different way of coping with bad news, particularly about health challenges. It's not uncommon for the newly diagnosed person to find himself or herself comforting a spouse or family member.

Two weeks later, Mona has the hysterectomy. James has managed to find additional help for the store and is planning to take care of Mona for the first few weeks of recovery. Mona has been given a six-week leave from work and gets through every day leading up to the surgery in a robot-like fashion. She has lost eight pounds in the weeks leading up to the surgery and hasn't been sleeping well. After five days, she's discharged and goes home to continue her recovery.

Mona is surprised by the overwhelming fatigue that she experiences. The incision on her abdomen is smaller than expected, but she's surprised by the amount of vaginal bleeding that she has. She can't recall being warned about this, and the irony is that it reminds her of her experience after the twins were born. The weeks of her recovery seem to alternatively fly and crawl by. Every day she can do a little more, but the smallest household tasks seem to overwhelm her. James goes back to working in the store full-time, and he tries to get back home once during the day to check on her. Most often he finds her sitting in front of the TV, deep in thought, but she won't share what she's thinking.

Dr. Katz Explains

Fatigue isn't uncommon after surgery, and it's often difficult to cope with the household chores and activities of daily life, even for the most efficient and energetic people.

Take-Away Points

- It's important to rest often, pace yourself, and allow sufficient time to recover both physically and emotionally.
- Accept help from family and friends; they may not do things exactly the way you do, but you need to conserve your energy for more important things than loading the dishwasher.
- There really is no timetable for recovery; it tends to happen in its own time, and fighting this usually results in even greater fatigue.

Uncertainty and Trepidation

Mona goes to her six-week check-up with some foreboding. While she's certainly feeling a lot stronger, she acknowledges to herself that she hasn't dealt with what will come next. She knows that further treatment is necessary, but she's not sure of the details or if she's even been told what the plan is. The gynecologist examines Mona and informs her that all is well with her healing and that she can now continue with life as before. Mona isn't sure if life ever will be the same but is feeling too overwhelmed to ask any questions. She's given a card with information about an appointment the following week at the cancer center where her radiation therapy will take place.

Dr. Katz Explains

This was a perfect opportunity for the doctor to give Mona specific information about her continued recovery and eventual return to normal functioning, including sexual activity. The physician's statement that she can "continue with life as before" is vague, and any patient who hears this might fear appearing stupid if she asks exactly what this means. In Mona's case, a valuable teaching opportunity has been lost, and this may lead to problems in the future.

Take-Away Point

- At the postoperative appointment, you should ask questions such as these.
  - What organs were removed during the surgery?
  - Are there any other changes to the area that might be affected by the surgery? (For example, it's normal for the upper third of the vagina to be removed during surgery for cervical cancer. This will shorten the vagina, and the woman needs to know that deep thrusting in the vagina during intercourse might be painful.)
  - What can be done if sex hurts? (The patient should be advised that changing sexual positions to ones where the woman controls the depth of penetration [woman on top or side by side] can be helpful.)

Mona attends the appointment with the radiation oncologist at the cancer center with trepidation. She hasn't done any research into radiation therapy and doesn't know what to expect. She is shown to an examination room; after a 10-minute wait, a tall man enters, introduces himself as the radiation oncologist, and, after a brief physical examination, explains what her treatment plan will be. Mona tries hard to concentrate on his words, but all she can think of is what radiation is going to be like and how she'll get through what lies ahead. The nurse returns with an armload of pamphlets, booklets, and videos. These are for Mona and James to review when they're ready, but the nurse suggests that they at least read one or two before her radiation treatments begin the following week. Mona is to have three sessions of internal radiation (high-dose brachytherapy).

Feeling Vulnerable

The next Monday morning, Mona and James reach the cancer center early and wait in silence for her appointment. Mona is taken into the brachytherapy suite while James waits in the waiting area. Staff asked if she wanted him to come in with her but she declined. She is positioned on the table with her legs placed into the stirrups, and the procedure begins. There seem to be a lot of people in the room. Mona assumes that they need to be there, but she feels exposed and vulnerable and closes her eyes to block them out. The nurses are efficient and caring; they explain everything to her and insert the applicator into her vagina with only minor discomfort. The radiation source is then placed in the applicator, and Mona has to lie very still for 15 minutes. The radiation source is removed, and she dresses and goes home.

Dr. Katz Explains

It's not uncommon for women to feel very exposed during medical procedures such as these. For the healthcare providers, treating women like Mona is routine, and they do their best to be professional and to respect the dignity of the patient. But for the patient, this is a new and unusual situation. Lying naked from the waist down in a room full of healthcare personnel can be a difficult experience, and many women respond in the same way as Mona does. They close their eyes and try to distance themselves from what is happening to their bodies.

This can have long-term consequences for the woman; by distancing herself from her body, she may be setting herself up for sexual difficulties if she can't find a way to reconnect with her body, specifically her genitals.

Take-Away Point

- When a woman is feeling vulnerable and disconnected from her body, she may begin to feel that her body is an object and not something that brings her pleasure. She may need to find ways to reconnect with her body as a source of pleasure. Some ways to do this include
  - Asking your partner or child to gently massage your hands or feet, back, or head and neck
  - Scheduling a regular massage, manicure, or hair appointment
  - Paying attention to the sensations as someone else cares for your body in a soothing, pleasurable manner.

At Last—The End of Treatment

Mona visits the cancer center two more times, and then her treatments are over. On her last day of treatment, the nurse gives her a plastic vaginal dilator with a sheet of instructions. Feeling exhausted and slightly embarrassed, Mona stuffs this into her purse, and when she gets home places it at the back of her closet.

Dr. Katz Explains

For women who have had internal radiation to the vaginal area, the long-term use of a dilator is recommended to keep the vagina open for both sexual activity and future pelvic examinations. After surgery, the vagina is shorter, and the radiation treatment poses the additional risk of changes to the lining of the vagina and actual shrinkage of the vagina itself. Using the dilator will prevent the walls of the vagina from sticking to each other, which would make intercourse painful and perhaps impossible and do the same for pelvic examinations.

Take-Away Points

- The dilator should be used three times a week for 10 minutes a session. Some women find it easier to start with a very small dilator and gradually increase the size.

- Most women find that using a lubricant with the dilator makes insertion more comfortable.
- Latex dilators are very comfortable to use and come in a range of different sizes and colors. They can be ordered from www.soulsourceenterprises.com.
- If and when intercourse is resumed, the use of a dilator can be stopped, but it's advised that vaginal dilation should occur three times a week for at least three years following radiation therapy.

Reestablishing Intimacy

Mona and James celebrate their wedding anniversary a few weeks after her radiation therapy is completed. As is their usual routine, they go out for dinner at a favorite restaurant. James seems quiet during dinner, but Mona doesn't say anything, and they go home early. Soon after, Mona is getting ready for bed. As she turns to switch off the bedside light, she is startled to feel James' arms around her waist. She gasps and feels herself pulling away and immediately feels guilty. She embraces him and they kiss and begin to touch each other. She is very tense, and James can sense that something is wrong. He pulls away from her, waiting for a response, and Mona moves to her side of the bed and turns over. They both lie awake in the dark for some time.

In the morning, Mona decides to raise the topic of what happened the night before. It's difficult for her to get the words out, but she manages to tell him that she feels guilty about what happened, but she's scared about making love again and doesn't know what to do. She tells him that when he touches her, she feels no physical excitement, and this is made worse by her fear of making love. James asks her if she's discussed this with any of her healthcare providers, and she admits that she's been reluctant to talk about it and doesn't know with whom to talk.

Dr. Katz Explains

Sexual arousal is a physical phenomenon where blood flow to the genitals increases in response to physical and mental stimulation, such as when a couple begins intimate touching. The blood flow to the vaginal walls leads to an increase in the amount of lubrication produced, and most women interpret this as a sign of arousal and readiness for intercourse. This physical response also is experienced as a pleasurable sensation indicating sexual excitement, which, in turn, increases the response. It's also affected by emotions, and anxiety can be a powerful barrier to feeling aroused. Mona has had surgery that may have destroyed or damaged some of the nerves supplying the vagina. Her vagina is shorter than it was before the surgery, so there's less vaginal tissue, and the part of the vagina that usually swells and increases in size during sexual excitement (the upper third of the vagina) has been removed.

In addition, internal radiation usually damages the tissues lining the upper part of the vagina, and less lubrication is produced. The tissues of the vagina can become inflamed and irritated following radiation therapy and may stick to each other. Scar tissue may form, and the vagina itself may become blocked. Bands of scar tissue may form; this is called *stenosis*.

Treatment Is Complete, But Issues Persist

Another month goes by, and Mona and James still haven't talked any further about what's happening in their now nonexistent sex life. Mona still hasn't contacted any of her healthcare providers to talk about this. She feels guilty about this a lot of the time but feels powerless to initiate any action. At her three-month follow-up appointment at the cancer center, the nurse asks Mona if she's using the dilator as instructed. Mona admits that she put it in the closet the day of her last brachytherapy treatment and hasn't looked at it since. As she talks about it, she starts to cry. The nurse sits and listens as Mona tries to explain her feelings. The nurse offers Mona a referral to a sex therapist, and Mona agrees half-heartedly.

Dr. Katz Explains

Some healthcare providers always ask about issues pertaining to sexuality, while others prefer to wait until the patient raises the issue. If you have a question or a concern, it's important to find the courage to ask because this may be the only way in which your concerns are discussed. Try not to be embarrassed; healthcare providers are used to answering questions like these.

Take-Away Point

- Mona needs to tell her healthcare providers what she experienced and ask for help in overcoming these difficulties. Some of the questions to ask include
  - Is there anything that can be done to help me relax before sexual activity?
  - How long can I expect to feel this way?
  - Is there some kind of lubricant I can use to help with my lack of natural lubrication?

Mona doesn't tell James about what happened when she talked to the nurse, and she also doesn't tell him about the appointment with the sex therapist. The tension between them is now palpable, and they avoid each other as much as possible. James has taken to staying up later than Mona, and she goes to bed early and falls asleep almost instantly.

Dr. Katz Explains

Mona and James are responding to this challenge in their lives in a fairly typical fashion. They have withdrawn from each other and are avoiding a confrontation about sex by avoiding each other at bedtime.

Denial and withdrawal is one way to deal with problems in a relationship, but it's not very effective and leads to the distance between the couple growing bigger. For some couples, the distance grows too large over time, and they're unable to repair the relationship.

Take-Away Points

- To deal with a lack of intimacy, set aside some time to talk about what is bothering you. You need to talk in "I" statements and talk only about your feelings.
- Don't place blame or suggest what the other person is thinking. Your partner should give you sufficient time to express yourself and then should be allowed to talk about his or her feelings. This is not easy.
- If necessary, seek out professional help, such as a trained counselor or religious adviser.

Finally Getting It All Out

Mona goes to the appointment with the sex therapist and is somewhat surprised to be greeted by a young woman, who ushers her into a pleasant office with leather furniture and sunlight streaming through large windows. For an hour, the therapist asks her questions about her experience being treated for cancer and her feelings about herself and her body. This is not at all what she expected, and she finds herself opening up and expressing herself quite freely about her feelings and emotions. The therapist tells Mona that she would like to meet with James alone and then with the two of them together.

Dr. Katz Explains

Many people aren't sure what to expect from a visit to a sex therapist. Mona's experience is somewhat typical; the therapist will ask about past experience and take a thorough history related to the presenting issue. It's also common for the therapist to want to talk to the partner/spouse separately and then to the couple together.

James Sees the Therapist

Mona isn't sure how to introduce the topic to James, but she feels so much better having talked to the therapist that she just blurts it out over dinner that evening. James is somewhat surprised that all of this has been going on without him knowing, but he's eager to find a way to resolve the situation and agrees to see the therapist at the earliest opportunity. His meeting with her also is pleasant. He is so happy that something may help to resolve what has become for him a very difficult situation that he talks a lot and repeatedly asks the therapist what she thinks will help. The therapist cautions him that it may take some time for Mona to feel ready to make love again and tells him that she wants to meet with them as a couple the following week.

Dr. Katz Explains

Finding solutions to sexual problems is not always a simple matter. While James is eager to fix this, the problems they are encountering have taken place over months, if not years, and "fixing" them may take some time. Not all men will seek professional help so willingly; many are afraid that seeing a therapist or counselor means that they are weak, and others may just think it is weird. Many people do not understand what goes on in counseling and may be fearful that they have to tell "secrets" about themselves. A good counselor will explain exactly what he or she does and what the boundaries are before starting any sort of work with couples or individuals.

The Couple's Turn

The following week, Mona and James go together to see the therapist. At this meeting, the therapist asks the couple to state their perspective on what has happened. Mona tearfully talks about feeling guilty for shutting James out. She explains that her body just doesn't feel like her own anymore, and she wishes it were different. She acknowledges that their distance from each other is difficult, but she isn't sure how to approach him after all this time. James describes feeling powerless to help Mona. He misses their lovemaking and feels tense and guilty when he masturbates. With some gentle probing from the therapist, Mona tells James that she can't imagine ever making love again. She has an image of her sexual organs as being shriveled and burned and she's afraid that if he touches her, it will hurt; but she's also afraid that if their lovemaking doesn't resume, he will leave her. She has tried using the dilator she was given, but it's too painful, and she's afraid to admit to the oncologist that she didn't comply with the prescribed treatment.

Dr. Katz Explains

It's often difficult to talk to a partner about sex and sexual problems. It is an emotionally charged topic that extends beyond the bedroom and into the person's self-confidence. As you can see from Mona and James, it extends into issues of abandonment and also touches on childhood issues, such as guilt about masturbation.

The therapist recommends that Mona and James practice sensate focus exercises (see Figure 2). These will help them regain some physical intimacy. She also suggests that Mona see the gynecologist again and ask about topical treatments for vaginal dryness.

Figure 2. How to Do Sensate Focus Exercises

In sensate focus touching exercises, partners take turns touching each other while following some essential guidelines. These exercises can be done by heterosexual as well as same-sex couples.

First, it's necessary to discuss some basic principles, which might include the following.
- Decide on the purpose of the exercise: Is it for the woman to experience pleasure or for the couple to eventually have intercourse again?
- Determine who will be the first giver.
- Establish whether you and your partner will be clothed or unclothed.
- Choose a location where you both will be comfortable, preferably not in bed.
- Dim the lights and play soft music you both enjoy.
- Use plenty of pillows or a comforter to ensure physical comfort.
- If you wish, use baby oils, scented oils, lotions, or powder.
- Tell the giver what feels good and what does not.

The exercises are divided into four progressive stages (see Figure 3). Master each stage before moving to the next. Repeat all previous stages each time. The pace depends on your progress and comfort. Consider these helpful suggestions.
- The toucher learns from the one being touched. The one being touched takes the partner's hand and controls the degree of pressure as well as the pattern and length of strokes. This is a learning experience for the partner who is doing the touching as well as the one who is receiving the touch.
- The learning hand of the toucher should not be his or her dominant hand. A right-handed person should use the left hand and left-handers, the right hand. This increases sensitivity.
- Do the exercises when you and your partner are rested and not pressed for time. Don't do the exercises after a heavy meal or when you've had a disagreement.
- At no time is there to be any attempt to have sexual intercourse, even if the male partner becomes sexually aroused. Intercourse should only be attempted at stage 4 (see stages below), if at all.
- After the session, you will want to discuss what you think you have accomplished and share positive as well as negative feelings with your partner.

Figure 3. Stages of Sensate Focus

The partners take turns being the giver and the receiver. Communication during the exercises is by guiding the hand of the partner giving the massage. Limit talking until after you complete the exercises.
- **First stage**: Limit touching and stroking to the areas of the body that are not sexually stimulating.
- **Second stage**: Touch, stroke, and explore the sensual responses of the entire body, including the breasts and genitals, without intent to bring about erection or vaginal lubrication.
- **Third stage**: Repeat the first two stages. Stroke the penis and clitoris and probe the vaginal opening with a finger. Note the occurrence of erectile and lubrication responses, if any. You don't have to discuss these, but concentrate on the sensations of arousal.
- **Fourth stage**: Repeat the first three stages. Caress and stimulate breasts and genitals. Use a lubricant, especially for the clitoris, the outer vulval lips, and the vaginal opening of the woman as well as for her partner with less than full erectile response. When the man's erection is firm enough to attempt penetration, the couple may want to insert the penis and feel it in the vagina. Or they may ignore this and just continue to pleasure each other without penetration.

Tips

If the intent is for the woman to experience pleasure, then whether her partner has an erection is not an issue. If the woman feels her partner is losing his erection, she can initiate pelvic movements until it returns. But this may not be the focus of the exercise for the couple. The exercise is never over as long as the couple feels comfortable with each other and is enjoying and savoring the good feelings.

The use of baby oil or body lotion is recommended for stages one and two of the sensate focus exercises.

A sexual lubricant is helpful during stages three and four when the genitals are touched. Recommended lubricants include Astroglide® (BioFilm, Inc.) and K-Y® (McNeil-PPC, Inc.).

Dr. Katz Explains

Over the past several months, Mona and James have grown distant from each other both physically and emotionally. Sexual activity is sometimes likened to the glue that holds relationships together; it's not that it's the most important aspect of the relationship, but when the closeness and connectedness that result from sexual activity are absent, the couple tends to drift apart. When this goes on for an extended period—and for each couple the definition of "extended" may be different—then the gap between them grows wider and deeper, and reconnecting is made even more difficult. Sensate focus exercises are a well-established method of helping couples who are experiencing sexual challenges to reconnect with each other.

Take-Away Points

- The gradual resumption of touching often is helpful to couples and allows them to once again establish physical closeness that may or may not include sexual intercourse.
- There is no ultimate goal, and the couple is encouraged to proceed with these exercises at their own pace with permission to remain at the level where they are most comfortable.

Mona and James: Gradually Reclaiming Their Sex Life

Mona received a prescription for an estrogen cream, which she inserts in her vagina three times per week. She is now using the dilator regularly and finds that since she has been using the estrogen cream, it's much easier to insert the dilator.

Mona and James continue to meet with the sex therapist for six months. They report that they have been practicing the sensate focus exercises on a regular basis, and while Mona remains fearful of penetrative intercourse, they are finding that they can both have their needs for sexual satisfaction met through genital and nongenital touching. The couple admits that they're closer now than they've ever been and are finding that they're talking to each other much more. And bedtime is no longer a challenge; they go to bed at the same time each night and are content to fall asleep in each other's arms.

Dr. Katz Explains

Mona and James in some ways are lucky; they've found a way of meeting their own sexual and emotional needs through nonpenetrative touching. Not all couples will be happy with this. Other couples will mourn the loss of their previous sex life and may prefer to avoid any and all sexual touching if they can't do it the way they did before.

Take-Away Points

- Sensate focus exercises can be helpful in providing an alternative to penetrative intercourse.
- Oral sex also can be a satisfactory alternative for some couples.
- Other couples find that "outercourse" works well. The woman sandwiches the man's penis between her thighs and the man thrusts as usual. Using lubricant on the thighs/penis makes this much easier and more pleasurable.

CHAPTER 6

Problems With Orgasm

It just doesn't feel the same . . . the fireworks are gone.

Treatment for cancer can affect one's ability to have an orgasm. There is no single reason for this. It may be that surgery has altered the anatomy of the sexual organs, or it may be something emotional after you've gone through the whole experience. Orgasms are partly physical but also have a large emotional and psychological component.

Many women have difficulty having orgasms. Some women have never had an orgasm and don't mind that; others struggle for years trying to find a way to have one. There are many books written to help women have orgasms, and many have been bestsellers. Some women can have an orgasm with masturbation but never with their partner. Others can only have orgasms with oral sex or if they use a vibrator.

In this chapter, you will read about Rosemary, who found that after treatment for bladder cancer, she could no longer have orgasms during sex with her partner. You will learn

- How to overcome physical and emotional challenges related to cancer
- How to enjoy a satisfying sexual life after cancer treatment.

Rosemary's Story

Rosemary is 63 years old and was diagnosed with bladder cancer a year ago. She'd noticed some blood in her urine but had ignored it for months, as she thought it was related to menopause even though she'd gone through it 10 years earlier. By the time she saw her primary care provider, the cancer was advanced, and she had to have extensive surgery followed by chemotherapy.

Dr. Katz Explains

Bladder cancer often presents with some blood in the urine. Sometimes it is in such minute quantities that the person doesn't notice. Treatment depends on the stage of the cancer; if caught early, surgeons may be able to remove the tumor only or surgery may not be needed at all. In Rosemary's case, the cancer was advanced, and she had to have extensive surgery as well as chemotherapy.

Practice Makes Perfect, Even in Marriage

Rosemary has been married to Mario for seven years. This is a second marriage for them both. She is divorced from her first husband, and Mario's wife died of breast cancer just six months before he met and married Rosemary. Mario has a large Italian family with many siblings to whom he is very close.

The marriage has been very happy for them both. Rosemary's first marriage was difficult, and she waited until her three children were settled in their own relationships before leaving her husband. Mario really struggled after his first wife died; they had no children, which was a source of great sorrow to them both, and her last year with breast cancer was long and painful. Mario and Rosemary met at the library and even though he was newly widowed, the attraction was instant, and they started dating and were soon married.

Mario was devastated by Rosemary's diagnosis. She found herself comforting and supporting him even when she had to make some difficult decisions about treatment. But she loves him, and that is how things go sometimes.

Dr. Katz Explains

It's not uncommon for someone newly diagnosed to find herself comforting and supporting loved ones. Everyone reacts to this news differently, and some people see cancer as a death sentence and are struck with grief at the news. If the person has lost someone else to cancer, as Mario had, it can be especially difficult to go through it again with a loved one. Today, the majority of those diagnosed with cancer go on to live for many years after their diagnosis and treatment. There are more than 10 million cancer survivors in the United States today, which is very different from even 20 years ago.

Surgery

Rosemary's treatment involved surgery to remove the bladder, part of the wall of the vagina, the uterus and ovaries, and part of the urethra, the tube through which urine flows to the outside. The surgeon then created a neo-bladder from part of the intestine to form a bag inside the body. The neo-bladder holds the urine that she passes in the normal manner but Rosemary also has to insert a rubber catheter into the neo-bladder to make sure that the bladder is completely empty. She does this in the bathroom and lets the urine flow into the toilet.

Dr. Katz Explains

Because Rosemary's cancer was found at a late stage, she had to have extensive surgery. A lot of tissue was removed during the surgery, and the surgeon used some of the tissue from the intestine to create a "new" bladder where urine can be stored inside the body rather than outside in a bag. Even though she can pass urine normally in the toilet, she has to also insert a catheter (a thin, flexible tube made out of a silicone material) into her new bladder to make sure that there's no urine left behind and that the bladder is totally empty. This is important to prevent urinary tract infections.

What She Remembered

She remembers the doctors and nurses explaining the seriousness of the surgery, but at the time she was so worried about Mario that she mostly nodded her head and did not ask any questions. She is a woman of deep faith and believed at the time, and still does, that God will take care of her and protect her.

Dr. Katz Explains

As you have read in the accounts of different people in this book, when people receive a cancer diagnosis, they often don't hear everything that's said. Sometimes it's because the person is so shocked because he or she did not expect it or perhaps because he or she starts thinking about what this means and how it will affect other people. Most people only remember 10% of what was said after they hear the words "You have cancer."

Support Comes From Different Places

Six weeks after surgery, Rosemary started her chemotherapy treatments. Mario found it difficult to accompany her to the cancer center; it reminded him of his first wife and her struggle, and even though that was almost eight years ago, he still could not bring himself to go with her. Fortunately, his siblings were able to help, and every day of her chemo treatments, one of her sisters-in-law sat with her. She is grateful for their presence in her life and loves them as if they were her own sisters. Rosemary has a big heart and was not upset that Mario couldn't go with her. In a way, she thought that her treatment was "women's business" and was happy to spend the time with whichever sister-in-law was there with her.

Family Sustenance

Rosemary was not well during the weeks of chemotherapy. She was exhausted most of the time and experienced sores in her mouth that made it impossible to eat much of anything. She lost a lot of weight on top of what she lost in the weeks after her surgery, when she had very little appetite. Mario's family loves to eat, and much of their family life revolves around meals and holidays. This is something that Rosemary loved, and she really enjoyed the hours spent with the other women talking and preparing and cooking huge family meals for the large extended family. The men would sit around while all this was happening, laughing and drinking the homemade wine that they made together in the late summer. But for most of the past year, Rosemary has not been able to fully participate in these activities. When she's been able to join them for Sunday lunch, she mostly sits and watches; her energy levels are not what they used to be, and she has no stamina. But she still feels included in the group of women.

Dr. Katz Explains

Surgery, itself, is very draining, and Rosemary had extensive surgery. Many people find that it takes a long time to fully recover. If they lost a lot of blood during the surgery, it may take a long while to regain an appetite for food, and not eating means you take even longer to feel better.

Some people get mouth sores when they have chemotherapy. The medications used in this treatment target cells in the body that divide quickly. This is what cancer does, and so the medication is designed to kill the cancer. Unfortunately, other cells in the body also divide quickly. These include the cells in the tissue lining the mouth and throat and also hair cells. That's why people who have chemotherapy often lose their hair and also get mouth sores.

You Can Learn New Tricks

For a long time she's wanted to ask her sisters-in-law about something really private that's causing her a lot of worry. Ever since her surgery, she and Mario have not had sex often, but when they do, she never has an orgasm. In fact, she feels almost nothing "down there." This is so different from what sex was like with Mario before the surgery. Something that really surprised her about Mario was how much he enjoyed sex and how much she enjoyed it with him. With her first husband, sex was almost nonexistent. And when it happened, it was over almost before she even really knew something was happening. She had nothing to compare it to; she'd married for the first time when she was 20 years old, and her first husband was the first man she had sex with. She sometimes thought that her three pregnancies were some kind of miracle.

When she married Mario, she was very shy and was quite nervous about what would happen in the bedroom. But Mario just swept her along with his great passion and love, and she was really amazed at her response. At the age of 56, she had her first orgasm, and this was like a revelation for her. For the first time in her life, she actually enjoyed the physical contact, and over the first six years of their marriage, sex was very important.

Since her surgery, she has been somewhat reluctant to have sex with Mario. Even though she misses it, the first time they had sex it hurt, and she's scared that it will hurt all the time. She's also scared that she'll leak urine during sex; this happened the first time they tried, and she was so embarrassed. Mario didn't seem to notice, but she did, and the memory hasn't left her. She remembers having to change the bed sheets, and she made Mario take a shower while she cried as she made the bed before they went to sleep.

Take-Away Points

- Urine is sterile and not harmful to either you or your partner.
- If you're concerned about odor, suggest that you and your partner take a bath or shower before sexual activity. This is also a good place to have sex, as any leakage will be hidden by the water. Just be careful about not slipping on the wet surface.
- Use a towel or plastic sheet on the bed to protect your linens.
- Self-catheterizing just before sexual activity can reduce the chances of leakage, as can restricting fluids for a couple of hours before sexual activity.
- If penetration causes pain deep in the vagina, it may mean that scar tissue has formed and you may need extra time and stimulation to get fully aroused, which will help to enlarge the vagina.

Dr. Katz Explains

After surgery like this, it's not unusual to have pain with intercourse. Some of Rosemary's vagina had been removed, and it's probable that her vagina is now shorter than it was before. The first time they have sex after surgery and chemotherapy, most women are a little tense, and this can also cause the muscles in the vagina to tense up and make penetration painful.

Fear of leaking urine is very real, too. For most of us, leaking urine is embarrassing. Many women who have this experience because of loose pelvic muscles suffer greatly; they wear pads all the time and are constantly changing them and washing themselves to control odor. When leakage happens during sex, it can really be troubling. It's no longer private, and you may think that your partner is going to be disgusted by this.

Where Did the Orgasms Go?

And since then, she has not had a single orgasm. Not even the hint of one. She's not talked to Mario about this; the last time they made love she pretended to have an orgasm. She felt really bad about this afterward, but he seemed so happy, and she didn't want to ruin the moment. The next time she faked it, too. And she felt even worse as she knew she was lying, which made her feel ashamed.

Dr. Katz Explains

Rosemary may not be having orgasms for a lot of reasons. First, there may be some nerve damage from the surgery affecting her sexual response. And it may be that she's nervous about having sex and anxious about having pain because this has happened before. The brain can really interfere with orgasms, and any worry you're having can affect the way you respond to your partner.

Take-Away Points

- Worrying about orgasms really doesn't help. It actually makes it harder because if you're worried, you're also tense, and tension and orgasms don't mix.
- Faking is not a good idea. It sends the wrong message to your partner, who thinks that he or she is doing what you need to be satisfied. So, your partner will continue doing what he or she thinks works, and you'll never get what you need!

Talking About Sex

She wants to talk to her sisters-in-law about this. When the women get together, they often talk about sex. This is a family where nothing's off limits, and she's learned a lot from these women, who range in age from 52 to 70 years. They all have the same zest for life as Mario even though three of them also are in-laws and married to Mario's brothers. One Saturday evening in late summer, she finds the courage to raise the topic.

In a small voice she tells them that things have been "different" since her treatment. The women are quiet for a few minutes when she finishes, and then Maria, the oldest of the sisters, hugs her and tells her that she understands. Maria had breast cancer five years ago, and just six months ago her husband of

49 years died after having a stroke. And the youngest sister reaches out a hand and tells Rosemary that she, too, has noticed a difference since she went through menopause. Soon they're all talking and listening to each other's stories. But as much as Rosemary's grateful for their support and understanding, she doesn't find much useful information from the discussion.

Dr. Katz Explains

It can be really helpful when you can share your concerns with friends or family members. For some of us, knowing that we're not alone brings comfort. But sometimes you need professional help because your friends and family may not know what to do to help you.

Seeking Help

Just admitting to someone else that she had a problem seemed to help Rosemary, and the next day she called her family physician to make an appointment to talk about it. Her physician's a much younger woman, but Rosemary feels at ease with her, and she was very helpful when Rosemary had mouth ulcers during chemotherapy. At her appointment, Rosemary rushes through her story. She talks very fast and very softly, and Dr. Samuels has to ask her a number of times to slow down or talk louder. Eventually she gets the whole story out: her body has let her down, she feels dead down there, she no longer enjoys sex, she's lied to Mario, and she doesn't know how to fix this.

Dr. Samuels starts at the beginning and takes a sexual history from Rosemary. And then she asks her patient what she remembers about the surgery and what parts of her body were removed. Rosemary looks surprised at this question. The surgery seems such a long time ago, and it was necessary to remove the cancer. Dr. Samuels examines Rosemary and even though everything seems normal, Rosemary points out that she can barely feel the doctor examining her. When Rosemary is dressed Dr. Samuels continues their conversation. She tells Rosemary that there may be many reasons why sex is now not the same as it was before. She draws a diagram on a piece of paper showing her patient exactly what was removed and where nerves and blood vessels had been destroyed. Rosemary absorbs all this in silence and does not ask any questions.

Dr. Katz Explains

Dr. Samuels is doing something really helpful for Rosemary. She's going over a lot of the same things that Rosemary was told before her surgery but just couldn't retain or remember. This is helpful so that Rosemary can learn about the physical basis of her problem and not assume that it's in her head.

Take-Away Points

- It's never too late to ask exactly what was removed during surgery or about the treatments you've had.
- Some of us are more visual than others, and a drawing can really help us understand what goes where and what happens when it's no longer there.

Broken Body

The next weekend she tells her sister-in-law Maria that she's a broken woman. In her words, she feels that she's no longer "whole" and that her "important parts" are missing. Maria's sympathetic but has no suggestions to offer. She does ask Rosemary if she asked Dr. Samuels for advice, and Rosemary has an idea: she'll see Dr. Samuels again and ask her what to do.

Dr. Katz Explains

Rosemary has taken what her physician explained and put her own spin on it. Dr. Samuels didn't talk about her as "being broken" or "not whole," but that's what Rosemary has taken from the conversation. It really doesn't matter what anyone says; what's important is what we take away from a discussion. In my practice, I often ask patients what they've understood before they leave. This gives me the opportunity to clear up misunderstandings or explain things again if I need to.

Missing Orgasms: Part 2

One week later, Rosemary once again is in Dr. Samuels' office. This time, she has a list of questions for her physician. Dr. Samuels asks Rosemary what her most important issue is. Rosemary replies it's her inability to have an orgasm and, related to that, her feelings of guilt about lying to Mario. Dr. Samuels once again explains why Rosemary may be having these problems with orgasm and gives Rosemary a book to read. She advises Rosemary to talk honestly to Mario and to do it before she's tempted to lie again about having an orgasm. Mario's going to be part of any solution Rosemary will find, and honesty is an important part of that.

Dr. Katz Explains

Sexual problems are always a couple's problem because the solution rests with both members of that couple. Unless your only sexual activity is masturbation, there should be another person with you to work things out.

The Book Recommends . . .

The book suggests that a woman who's having problems having orgasms should use a more intense form of stimulation, such as a vibrator. Rosemary shakes her head when she reads this; she cannot imagine where she would get such a thing, and, anyway, it just seems unnatural. But she leaves the book lying on the chair where Mario is likely to see it.

Dr. Katz Explains

Many women, particularly those in their middle years or older, have some difficulty with the idea of using a vibrator. It's how we've been socialized over the years and the messages we've learned about pleasure and sex and how women ought to be. There is nothing unnatural about finding ways to experience pleasure. Many of us read recipe books and magazines about food so that the food we prepare looks and tastes great. Why is there such a difference with sexual pleasure?

Mario Time

Mario sees the book on the chair and asks Rosemary where she got it. Rosemary blurts out that Dr. Samuels gave her the book, and she wants to try something the book talks about. Mario's a bit confused but lets her talk. She tells him that the surgery took away things from her and that she doesn't enjoy sex as much as she used to. Mario nods and motions for her to continue. He's noticed that things are different—you'd have to be blind not to—but once again he was influenced by his first wife's experience with cancer, and after her diagnosis, they never had sex again.

Dr. Katz Explains

Our partners usually notice things even if we think they don't. But this is a difficult topic, and Mario had previous experience with this and has just reacted the same way he did all those years ago. Rosemary has come a long way; she's telling him things honestly and opening up about a difficult subject.

Spilling the Beans

By this time, Rosemary's in tears. But she moves away when Mario reaches out to hold her. She wants to tell him everything now and doesn't want to be distracted. He stays where he is although every cell in his body tells him to reach out and hold her. She tells him everything in one long burst—how she'd lied about having an orgasm the last few times they had sex and that she feels nothing when they're having intercourse. She tells him that Dr. Samuels gave her the book to read, and the book suggests some things that may improve the situation.

Mario listens and then hugs her. He tells her he's not angry that she lied to him about the orgasms; he knew from her response to him in bed that it was different for her. He's just sad that she felt she had to lie. And he tells her that he wants to fix what's wrong and will do anything to make things as good as the way they were before.

Dr. Katz Explains

This is the best possible scenario that could happen for Rosemary. She's been honest, and Mario is accepting and wants to be part of the solution. He's honest with her, too; he tells her that he's known all along that something wasn't right and acknowledges that he's sad that she lied to him. This open communication means that, in the future, they'll be able to talk about anything because nothing bad happened this time.

Take-Away Points

- Honesty is really the best policy. Lying creates barriers that are difficult to overcome.
- Your partner wants you to be happy and satisfied, and if he or she knows there's a problem, he or she will work hard to fix it—if you let your partner.

A Man of Action

Mario opens the book and starts to read. Rosemary watches in silence as his eyebrows go up and down and a small smile occasionally flits across his face. After 20 minutes, her patience runs out; she moves next to him and they read together. He asks her if they should go to the sex store and buy a vibrator. Rosemary's unsure and hesitates, telling him to finish reading before making a decision. He completes that section, puts down the book, and announces that they are going to the drugstore right away. Rosemary's quite shocked, but when she looks at his face and sees the big grin, she also smiles and they both start to laugh. She's not sure why they're going to the drugstore, but he looks so happy she thinks she'll just indulge him.

Mario explains on the way to the drugstore that the book said that a massager usually used for the relief of back pain can be used "down there." He thinks that's a pretty good place to start, so off they go to buy one. The drugstore has a large range of massagers with photos on the box of men and women using the device on their backs and shoulders. Mario makes a joke about the other kinds of photos that they could put on the box, and Rosemary blushes.

Dr. Katz Explains

While an adult novelty store or online sex store will have a large range of vibrators in different shapes and sizes, most of them with really interesting names, a wand-type massager from the drug or department store can do exactly the same thing.

Trial and Error

They go home, and Mario is eager to try out the massager. He is met with a stony stare from Rosemary. It is 11 am and she has things to do around the house. Over the next week, Mario suggests every day that they give the massager a try. And every day, Rosemary makes an excuse. Even though she senses his eagerness and now his frustration, she is just not ready. She tries not to think about it, but every time she sees Mario's face, the pressure rises, and she feels bad.

Dr. Katz Explains

Everyone has a different way of doing things, and Rosemary and Mario are perfect examples of this. Now that they have purchased the massager, Mario wants her to use it; she needs to take her time. Although she went along with his plan to buy it, that does not mean she is ready to use it. This becomes a source of tension between them, and the pressure builds every day.

Fighting Words

One day they argue. It's a big fight, and it's as if all the pressure and pain of the last few months comes spilling out. Rosemary tells him that she is feeling pressure, and he tells her that he feels like he's going to explode from lack of sex. She yells back that he can just take care of himself, and as the words come out of her mouth, she realizes what the solution is. She needs to use the massager on her own. She needs to take care of herself, just to see if it works and what her response is. Mario's not sure what happened; one minute they were fighting, and the next minute she had kissed him on the cheek and the argument was over.

Dr. Katz Explains

Rosemary has come to an important realization: trying a vibrator may be best done alone. This makes perfect sense. By trying it without a partner present, you take away a lot of pressure. This is something new for Rosemary, and she's not yet sure if she'll like it or if it'll work. By experimenting on your own, you have some freedom to get used to it and to find out what works for you without trying to please someone else.

Going It Alone

The next afternoon, Mario goes to play cards with his friend. Rosemary decides that it's now or never, and she gingerly takes the massager out of its box. It is wand-shaped with a soft rubber knob on the end. There's a speed control switch that has variable settings from low to high. She takes it into their bedroom and plugs it into the wall outlet. She's not sure what to do with it and starts by holding it over her left shoulder, just like the photograph on the box. The sensation is pleasant, and she moves the speed control until she finds a speed that is comfortable. After five minutes she decides to try it "down there." At first she's unsure where to put it. Should she undress? What speed should she use? How is she supposed to know what to do? She lies down on the bed and holds the massager over the front of her genital area. She can feel the vibrations in her pubic bone, but the sensation is neither pleasant nor unpleasant, and it is certainly not sexually exciting. She moves the wand around a bit and suddenly she feels it, a definite tingle. She holds the massager very still over the spot, not trusting herself to move it and change the sensation.

She is surprised at how good the sensation feels, and within three minutes she has an orgasm. It's definitely an orgasm although it feels different from the ones she used to have with Mario. But she had an orgasm. She can't wait to tell Mario and does so as soon as he walks in the door. He was pretty happy, as he won $13 at cards, and tells her that her news is like winning the jackpot.

Dr. Katz Explains

Rosemary has experienced what millions of women the world over know: it's quite easy to have an orgasm with a vibrator. These devices provide intense stimulation just where it's needed. It's something that the woman can control and doesn't need to go into a sex store to buy (if that's a problem for you). You can find them anywhere personal grooming items are sold.

Take-Away Points

- Wand massagers produce strong vibration. This may be too intense for some women.
- If it's too intense, try looking for a smaller battery-operated vibrator in a sex store or online. These produce less intense sensation but still do the trick.
- You can easily take the wand massager on vacation with you. Airport security will just think you have back problems.
- Experiment with different speeds if the device has this option; slower may be better than faster for you, or the other way around.

Getting Over the Fear

Mario is now eager to try it again, but Rosemary's still not sure how she feels about having to use it. It still feels unnatural to her. She goes to see Dr. Samuels again; her previous advice and the book have been helpful, and she just wants someone to tell her that this is okay. Dr. Samuels is pleased to hear that Rosemary is doing something about her problem. She assures her that many women use vibrators and that for some women, it is the only way that they can have an orgasm. She makes some suggestions to Rosemary that may help her incorporate the massager/vibrator into her and Mario's love life.

Dr. Katz Explains

Doing things differently is not easy, especially in one's sex life. Most of us have been doing the same things with the same person for years, and it works. Moving outside of your comfort zone really is challenging, and it helps to have a sense of humor when experimenting.

Try a Little Patience

Rosemary tells Mario exactly what Dr. Samuels has told her. She also tells him that this is difficult for her and that he needs to be patient with her.

His only reply is to wrap her in his arms and tell her that he loves her and that she's made his life wonderful.

It's Now or Never

That weekend, Rosemary locks the front door of their house, turns off the ringer on the phone, and invites Mario to have a shower with her. She's still concerned that she'll leak urine during sex, and even though he says it doesn't bother him, he's learned to do what she says, which makes things easier. They use the massager/vibrator during foreplay and for the first time in ages, Rosemary feels aroused and ready for penetration. She's still a little nervous that it'll hurt, but this is the first time in a long while that she's felt this aroused, and she just goes with the feelings. When his penis enters her, she holds her breath but it's not painful. Mario is finished just a few minutes later. He lies down next to her and asks her how it was for her. Rosemary is just about to say "fine" when she remembers that she has to tell the truth and admits that while she felt aroused and the actual intercourse felt pleasant, she did not have an orgasm. Mario reaches over and picks up the massager/vibrator. He asks her if he can use it on her, and she closes her eyes and nods in agreement. She's tense, afraid, and embarrassed. She needs to guide his hand so that the vibrations are in the right spot. It once again takes only a few minutes and she has an orgasm. Just the look on Mario's face is enough to make her cry. He's so happy that she's had an orgasm, and it really was not that bad. Perhaps she could get used to this after all.

Dr. Katz Explains

Mario and Rosemary have succeeded in changing their usual routine and making it work. She did all the right things in preparation for this; she locked the door and turned the ringer off on the phone to ensure privacy and uninterrupted time for them. She took a shower and included Mario; this increased the confidence in her personal hygiene, which allowed her to relax. They used the massager as part of foreplay, and she tuned in to the sensation and found that she was aroused. Perhaps most importantly, she was honest with Mario about not having an orgasm from intercourse and allowed him to once again incorporate the massager/vibrator into their sexual activity. This produced the orgasm that was important for them both and has set the stage for other satisfying encounters in the future.

CHAPTER 7

Painful Sex

Sex isn't supposed to hurt.

Pain during sex comes as a shock to most women. They may feel pain at the entrance to the vagina with the touch of a partner's hand or when penetration occurs. They also can experience it with thrusting in the vagina or with orgasm. This pain and the memory of the pain can become a strong deterrent to future sexual activity.

There are many reasons why women experience pain during sexual activity. The most common reason is the drying of the tissues of the vagina and vulva because of the lack of hormones that normally keep the tissues moist or from damage to the blood supply of those tissues. Surgery may have altered the structure of the vulva and vagina. There may be internal or external scar tissue that prevents relaxation and stretching of the area.

Whatever the reason, the end result is that a once-pleasurable experience becomes a source of pain, which is not only physical but also can become emotional. Pain with sexual activity tends to create a cycle of fear and anticipation of pain that causes muscles to tense up, which then causes more pain. This cycle of pain can be difficult to break because the mind is powerful, and memories linger.

This chapter tells the story of Deb and Brent, a young couple who are struggling to cope with the aftereffects of radiation treatment for the anal cancer that Deb was diagnosed with. In this chapter, you'll learn

- How some women respond to radiation treatment in the genital area
- Why treating the mind as well as the body is important
- Why local hormone treatment can help with genital pain.

Deb's Story

Deb, 36, and Brent, 37, have been together for 15 years. They are both children of hippies from the '60s; they never quite got around to getting married. They live on a small island off the coast of Vancouver; both their fathers were draft dodgers and moved to Canada to avoid the Vietnam War. They married Canadian women and stayed and raised their families. Brent is a carpenter and earns enough from working for friends and neighbors to maintain their small farm on the island, where they raise goats for milk and grow their own vegetables. Deb raised their two girls and home-schooled them until they reached their early teens; they now attend junior high school on a neighboring island. Deb isn't sure what she wants to do now that the girls are at regular school.

While she's in Victoria doing some shopping, she decides to see her nurse practitioner for a check-up. She's embarrassed when she realizes it's been four years since her last Pap test. The nurse practitioner does her Pap smear but also does a rectal examination; she explains that she does this to feel the posterior surface of the uterus. Deb feels some pain when the nurse practitioner's finger passes through her anus. The nurse practitioner frowns as she's doing this, and Deb's a bit alarmed. She's told that there's something that just doesn't feel right. The nurse practitioner can feel something in a small area on the wall of anus and wants Deb to have a biopsy. This is done that afternoon because Deb has to travel back to her small farm on the island and doesn't want to have to stay overnight if she can help it.

Dr. Katz Explains

It's not unusual for a pelvic examination to include a rectal examination because this is the only way that the practitioner can feel both sides of the uterus. A mass or growth in the anus may indicate something suspicious; in this case, the nurse practitioner is concerned about the possibility that Deb has cancer.

Biopsy Blues

That afternoon, she sees a general surgeon in the same building, and he does a biopsy of the anal tissue. Deb's in shock—she just came in for a routine Pap test—and she takes the bus to the ferry and travels home, deep in thought. She hasn't told Brent about what happened in Victoria; he had his cell phone turned off, and anyway, she wants to sort the whole thing out in her head before she can tell anyone. He's asleep by the time she gets home, and she tells him over breakfast the next morning after she'd had a sleepless night.

Brent is shocked and also saddened that she had to go through this all alone. But he has an optimistic nature and assures her that everything will be okay. Three weeks later, there is a message on the answering machine for Deb to call the nurse practitioner as soon as possible. She waits for the next day to call; she needs to gather her thoughts and prepare for what the news may be.

Bad News and More Bad News

The nurse practitioner tells her the biopsy results show that she has stage I anal cancer and needs to be seen at the cancer center. The nurse practitioner has made the appointment already for the following Thursday and tells Deb that she can expect to be there all day as she will need blood tests and a CT and also to see the cancer specialist. Deb asks what kind of treatment she is likely to have and is told that anal cancer generally is treated with chemotherapy and radiation but that sometimes surgery may be necessary.

She travels back to Victoria the next Thursday, her heart full of fear and prayers. Brent wanted to come with her, but he has a big project going, and they both agree that he needs to move forward on that work as she will need him to come with her to other appointments in the future. She's not told anyone else about this diagnosis; she wants to learn more before telling the girls; in any case, she just can't get the words out about this yet.

Dr. Katz Explains

Anal cancer, like any other cancer, is treated according to the stage and grade of the cancer. Stage I anal cancer means that the cancer is quite small, less than 2 cm. Usually, surgery is performed for a stage I anal cancer, but if the cancer is close to the anal sphincter, the muscle that keeps the anus closed, surgery may damage that muscle, and radiation and chemotherapy are the alternative treatments.

The Treatment Plan and People

Deb sees the radiation oncologist at this first visit. He tells her that a team of specialists has reviewed her biopsy results and feels that radiation and chemotherapy is the optimal treatment for her. He also tells her that she'll need five weeks of radiation and also will have chemotherapy during the first and last week of radiation. He then introduces Deb to Pam, the nurse who works with him and who's responsible for the educational needs of all patients having radiation treatment as well as for providing ongoing support throughout the treatment phase.

How Much Can One Woman Take?

Pam can see how overwhelmed Deb is at this point. She offers her some juice, and they go into a conference room to talk some more. Pam asks Deb about her family and what plans need to be made, as she's going to need daily radiation treatments for five weeks. Deb looks shocked; even though she heard the words "radiation therapy," she had just not realized the logistics of this and hadn't even thought what this would mean for her daily life. She tries to think about how this will change her life. But she can't seem to formulate any intelligent thoughts on the topic and just stares at the table, unable to speak.

Pam is concerned about her; she seems so alone, and this is a lot to cope with. She has an appointment for her CT scan in the early afternoon, and it's now almost lunchtime. Pam asks Deb if she would like some company for lunch and walks with her to the coffee bar on the main floor, where they each buy a sandwich and find a table to sit. Pam is good at this; she sits quietly and waits for Deb to speak or ask a question. Deb picks at her sandwich and sips from her bottle of juice. Eventually she asks a question: "Will I survive this?" Pam uses this as an opportunity to talk to Deb about how this cancer has been found really early and that she has every hope of a good outcome. She briefly mentions that before she starts her treatments, they will have to talk about side effects.

Dr. Katz Explains

Coming to terms with having cancer and the different kinds of treatments and how they will affect your life and daily activities is overwhelming. Besides bringing someone with you to appointments to help you keep track of information, it is really helpful if you have a contact person who is a trained health professional to help you in this journey.

Take-Away Points

- It is very helpful to have a trained professional to help you negotiate the complex healthcare system.
- Fears about survival often are at the forefront of your concerns and may influence treatment choices.
- If you are the kind of person who likes percentages and numbers, ask about probabilities for survival. But if numbers confuse you, tell the healthcare team that you don't want to hear numbers and would prefer another way of receiving information that is meaningful to you.

Making Plans

Deb has her CT scan and once again takes the bus and then the ferry home. She's exhausted and crawls into bed without talking to Brent, who came in late from work. A few days later she gets a phone call from Pam, who tells her that the CT was normal and that her radiation will start three weeks from that day. She suggests that Deb bring her husband with her to the cancer center for the start of radiation therapy. She asks Deb if she has managed to arrange a place to stay in Victoria when she has her treatments, and Deb admits that she's just been too tired and depressed to do anything about it. She does have a friend who has a sister in Victoria, and she plans to speak to her soon, and perhaps she can stay with her.

The next day she visits her friend and tells her what's happening. Before she can even ask about staying with her friend's sister, her friend gets up to call her sister; within just a few minutes, Deb has a place to stay in Victoria. The house is on a

Take-Away Points

- Having a support network is so important, and friends and family really do want to help.
- Telling people about your cancer should be on a "need-to-know" basis, and only you know who needs to be told.
- Telling teenage children about your cancer may be easier when you have a treatment plan and a start date. This gives them something concrete to focus on and may help them cope with their fears.
- Your cancer center should have resources (e.g., books, videos) about this. Support groups for teens whose parents have cancer also are available (see www.cancercare.org).

direct bus route to the cancer center, and there is room for Brent as well. Deb sighs with relief; she'd been putting off even thinking about this, and in just a few minutes, a significant challenge has been solved. The next challenge is to tell her teenage daughters—something that she's been dreading. But they need to know, and now that she has a start date for her treatment, she has to do it. They will be home over the weekend, and she'll prepare to tell them at some point during that time.

Preparing for Treatment

Deb manages to get through the next few weeks. The girls took the news badly, and she spent hours comforting them and assuring them that everything would be okay. She hopes that she actually believes that herself. Brent continues to work long hours to complete the project he is working on. Pam, the nurse from the cancer center, had sent her a large envelope with reading material, but Deb hasn't been able to bring herself to read any of it.

The day before her first radiation treatment, Deb and Brent make the journey to Victoria. They meet once again with the radiation oncologist and also with Pam. Pam takes them to see the chemotherapy area where Deb will receive her treatments, and she meets one of the nurses there, who shows them around. Just seeing the area as well as the many patients sitting in large chairs with IV bags above their heads scares Deb. But she's glad to see it before she starts her treatments there.

Her accommodations at her friend's sister's home are perfect. She has a room at the back of the house with a window that overlooks a lovely garden. Heather, her host, is a teacher and has a calm demeanor. She gives Deb a key to the house and shows her around the kitchen and living areas. Deb once again is overwhelmed, this time with the generosity of a stranger who has opened her home to her and relieved her of another burden.

A Bright White Light

The next day, Deb arrives early for her first radiation treatment. She is shown to a small changing area and is told to remove all her clothes, including underwear. She is then escorted to one of the treatment rooms. It is large and cold with a very big machine in the middle. The radiation therapist explains to her that this is the machine out of which the radiation will be generated. There are a number of people in the room; she guesses they must be staff because they're all wearing scrubs and name tags. She's helped onto the table, and then her legs are placed in stirrups. She feels herself starting to shake, and her head starts to spin. She had just not expected this. It doesn't get much better. A bright white light is aimed at her genitals and she lies there, completely exposed. The same people are still in the room. They seem to be doing all sorts of things all around her. She lies there with tears falling down her cheeks and onto the pillow. Someone with a soft voice asks her to move down a bit on the table. Deb keeps her eyes closed and does as she's asked. The voice tells her that they're all going to leave the room, she's going to hear and feel the machine move around her, and that the treatment will be over in about 12 minutes. And that's what happens.

Dr. Katz Explains

Many people are not prepared for exactly what will happen during treatment. Deb is shocked when she has her first radiation treatment and is physically exposed, the privacy of her person, literally stripped away. Lying on the table like that with her most private parts exposed is a traumatic experience. Could this have been done differently? Certainly the staff could have explained what was going to happen, and at the least they should have covered her with a sheet. In the busyness of routine work, they overlooked something very important: This experience is anything but routine for the patient, and it is critical for staff to remember that.

Take-Away Points

- It's important that you are as well-prepared as possible for your treatment. If you are given written material, try to read it as it likely contains useful information.
- Ask for a tour of the treatment facilities so that you can have a picture of where you will be. This can help ease some anxiety when you start treatment.

And the Beat Goes On . . .

Every weekday for five weeks, Deb comes to the cancer center and endures the same treatment. During the first week, she has chemotherapy every day, and it goes quite well. She doesn't like being poked with needles every day, but because she's having only two weeks of chemotherapy, the oncologist decided not to insert a central line. She has some nausea in the first week, but her hair doesn't fall out.

But the worse thing is the radiation every day. She gets through it by closing her eyes and thinking about the beach near their farm. She tries to ignore the technicians and therapists that walk around the room as she lies on the table, her legs in the stirrups and the bright white light shining on her genitals. She tries to imagine the waves breaking over the sand in the early morning light with a fine misty rain falling from the steel-gray skies. She goes home every Friday afternoon on the ferry and stays until Monday morning, when she once again takes the ferry to Victoria. She feels welcome in Heather's home but tries to keep out of her way when she's there. She's feeling quite tired and spends most afternoons and evenings reading or watching TV. She goes to sleep early after talking to Brent, who's still really busy with projects.

Take-Away Points

- It's important to find a way to cope with different aspects of the treatment.
- Many people find that relaxation recordings, self-hypnosis, inspirational music, or readings help them get through the more unpleasant parts of treatment.
- Taking care of oneself is just as important as taking medication or any other form of treatment; listen to your body and rest and eat when your body tells you it's time.

Dr. Katz Explains

Deb is using an essential coping technique to get through the experience; she is disassociating from the physical experience to minimize the trauma. She also is experiencing a common side effect of radiation: fatigue. But she seems to be taking good care of herself, and perhaps staying at a stranger's house is a good thing; she is able to relax instead of trying to fulfill her usual role as she would have had she been in her own house.

Suffering the Side Effects

By the second week of treatment, she's experiencing a lot of pain in the anal area. She was told to expect this, but she didn't anticipate that it would be this bad. Pam keeps contact with her and gives her some cream to use to protect the delicate skin and mucous membranes. But the breakdown of tissue continues, and by the fourth and then the fifth and last week of radiation treatment, she's in severe pain and finds it really difficult to sit for any length of time. Her chemotherapy treatments are draining. She has to sit on a special cushion to take the pressure off her bottom, and on the second to last day of treatment, she notices a foul-smelling odor and discharge coming from her vagina.

Dr. Katz Explains

Because the vagina and rectum/anus are so close together, radiation to the anal area will also expose the posterior vaginal wall to damage from the radiation. Tissue breakdown is quite common with radiation, and some women may develop a passage between the two when the tissues break down. This may lead to feces leaking into the vagina, which is difficult to cope with. Even if this does not happen, when tissue damage occurs, the dead cells of the vagina will pass to the outside of the body; this results in vaginal discharge that can smell bad.

Take-Away Points

- Damage from radiation tends to occur in the last weeks of treatment because the damage is cumulative, meaning that it occurs after repeated exposure to radiation.
- Report anything out of the ordinary to your health-care provider.
- Even if your healthcare providers tell you that what you are experiencing is normal, it is better to tell them than to ignore something that may need to be treated.

Could Things Get Any Worse?

This is the last straw for her, and she calls Pam early in the morning in great distress. She sees the radiation oncologist, who examines her and tells her that she's developed a breakdown in the tissue of the vagina where it shares a common wall with her rectum. She will need to have special packing placed in the vagina every day to help this heal and to prevent infection. She's at a loss to try and figure out how she's going to manage this on her own. Pam tells her to ask Brent to do it. Once again Deb is speechless; how can he possibly do this? She's given a large shopping bag full of supplies and once again takes the ferry home. She's exhausted and nauseous and terrified, so much so that she hardly acknowledges that her treatment is over.

Welcome Home

Back at home Brent has prepared a special celebration dinner. There are wild flowers in a vase, candles, and their best dishes set out on the table. She can smell the pasta sauce on the stove, and she knows that Brent has come home early to do this for her. But all she wants to do is crawl into her own bed and pull the covers over her head.

Later that night while they are lying in bed, she tells Brent about this latest complication, and as she expected, he takes it in stride and tells her he will do whatever he can to help her. The next morning he does just that; after her shower, she finds him emptying the shopping bag and sorting the items into piles. In a matter-of-fact manner, he gets her to lie on the edge of the bed and carefully pushes the packing coated in antibiotic cream into her vagina. Deb apologizes over and over the entire time he's doing this. He doesn't answer her until he's done, when he tells her that it doesn't matter to him. He even makes an attempt at a joke—he tells her that he's good with his hands—and she manages a small grimace in response.

Getting Better

After four weeks of daily dressings, she feels much better. She has a follow-up appointment at the cancer center, and the radiation oncologist tells her that her vagina has healed well and that she can now go back to "regular activity." She laughs in her head at this. What is normal now?

Dr. Katz Explains

The body has an amazing ability to heal, and people have an equally wonderful ability to cope with whatever life throws at them. Brent was able to help Deb with the packing and was happy to help her even though this was difficult for Deb to accept.

When Sex Hurts

One month later, Deb and Brent celebrate their anniversary. They have a lovely dinner at home that they both prepared. That night, for the first time since her diagnosis and treatment, they plan to have sex. She's nervous, but physically she's feeling so much better. She's had two glasses of wine and yet she just can't relax properly, and when Brent tries to insert his penis in her vagina, she pulls away with a small cry of pain. Brent stops immediately, turns on the bedside light and asks her what's wrong. "It hurts, it hurts" is all she can manage. Brent holds her until she eventually falls asleep.

Dr. Katz Explains

Nerves can play havoc with one's vagina. Deb obviously is anxious about how things will go after all this time and the treatment and complications she experienced. Experiencing pain with penetration can lead to long-lasting problems because you anticipate the pain every time, and your muscles tense up, which then contributes to the pain.

Take-Away Points

- Remember the relaxation exercises you used to relax before a treatment? These can help with relaxing before sex, too.
- Wine may relax you, but it can also remove your ability to focus and control your feelings. It also may affect pain receptors, so use with caution.

The Power of Remembering

The next day, she calls the nurse practitioner again and asks to see her. She tells her what happened the night before and asks her to check what is going on "down there." Deb once again travels to Victoria.

Before doing the examination, the nurse practitioner asks Deb to tell her about the treatment and how she felt during all that. Deb tells her about the breakdown of tissue and how Brent had to pack her vagina with dressings every day for weeks. She talks about lying on the table for the radiation treatments and the bright white light shining on her genitals. Everything comes out in a jumble of words and tears and hiccups as the tears pour down her cheeks.

The nurse practitioner just sits and listens. At the end of her story, Deb sits very quietly, obviously drained from the outpouring of emotion. The nurse practitioner tells Deb that she needs to get some help dealing with this experience and suggests that she see a psychologist who specializes in helping people who have experienced some sort of trauma. Deb thinks this is a little strange—she had cancer, not a trauma—but she trusts her and agrees to the referral.

Take-Away Points

- Many different kinds of healthcare providers are available to help those who are experiencing challenges during and after treatment.
- Accept all the help that is offered, even if you're not sure it's going to help. Going to one appointment is not all that difficult, and you may be surprised at what you learn.

Dr. Katz Explains

Deb is displaying signs of having gone through a traumatic experience. We all react differently to the same situations, and Deb found the radiation treatments themselves to be difficult, and then she also had some complications that prolonged her recovery. Most women who have gone through the same thing could benefit from some help making sense of it all and dealing with lingering feelings.

Getting Help

Three weeks later, Deb and Brent go to the first appointment. The psychologist is a young woman with a big smile and a soft voice. She asks Deb to tell her the whole story. By the end of the story, Deb once again is exhausted. Brent has listened attentively, and he has a deep frown on his sunburned face. Before the psychologist gets a chance, Brent asks Deb why she didn't tell him about the radiation treatments at the time; she'd never described in detail how she felt with the bright white light and the people in the room. Deb answers that she just needed to get through it, and there was nothing he could do about it anyway.

The psychologist asks some additional questions, and Deb answers them while Brent looks troubled. He interrupts the conversation between Deb and the psychologist and tells Deb that he feels so bad for trying to have sex on the night of their anniversary and that he didn't mean to hurt her. Deb tries to reassure him but then stops herself and tells him that, truthfully, she cannot imagine ever making love again, and she is not sure why he still wants to do that after everything he has done to her.

The psychologist stops them at that point and asks them to think about the words that Deb has just used; she used the words "after everything that you did **to** me." The couple is quiet for a long moment, and they realize something they'd not seen before. They start to talk to each other, explaining feelings and thoughts and interpretations of their behavior over the past months. They've had a breakthrough in a very short time.

Dr. Katz Explains

Even though Brent did everything he could to help Deb during that time, her response is her own and is neither right nor wrong. In this case, she felt as if he was doing something *to* her, and not *for* her, which many of us would think. She was very traumatized by what had happened, and because they'd not really talked about it at all, they both held many assumptions that were perhaps contributing to their feelings.

Dealing With the Aftermath

Deb still has a physical problem; her vagina and anal area have been damaged by the radiation, and even though the radiation oncologist seemed satisfied with her progress, she has pain, and sex is just not possible even though she wants to re-connect with Brent in this way. She calls Pam, the nurse who was so helpful during her treatments. Pam organizes a visit to a gynecologist, and after a brief examination, the gynecologist tells Deb that she's going to need to use a dilator regularly to prevent her vagina from closing as a result of the damage from the radiation.

This seems like a simple solution, and over the next few weeks Deb uses the dilator every other night. She doesn't like using the dilator and worries that Brent will walk into the room and see her. He takes great care to leave her alone when he knows she is in their room, but he wishes he could help her in some way. He suggests that they go back to see the psychologist; he tells Deb that he found it useful to talk in her presence, and he thinks there are still things that they need to sort out. To his surprise, she agrees without an argument and the next day schedules another appointment.

Dr. Katz Explains

When tissue has been damaged, it often exudes fluid as part of the healing process. In the vagina, this fluid can lead to the walls of the vagina sticking together. Scar tissue also develops, and this, too, can shorten and narrow the vagina. The dilators will help to keep the vagina open, which is important not only for sex but also for any future pelvic exams.

Take-Away Points

- If you've had radiation to the genital area, it's important to follow instructions for dilator use. Using the dilators can really help to prevent permanent changes to the vagina.
- It's also a good idea to take some time by yourself to feel what is happening "down there"; what you may think your vagina is like may not be accurate, and feeling yourself can help.

Deb Draws a Mental Picture

The second time they meet with the psychologist, they are both less nervous. Brent was surprised that he was able to talk so openly in her office before and hopes that the same thing will happen this time. The psychologist asks how they've been doing and what's brought them back. Brent tells her that even though they talked a lot during their last appointment, at home, Deb is withdrawn and doesn't share her feelings with him. Deb bristles at this. In a shaky voice she tells him that she hates what's happened to her body and having to use the dilators, and she just doesn't understand how he could still desire her sexually after everything that's happened.

The psychologist asks Deb to describe how she sees her body and, in particular, how she sees her genitals. Deb thinks for a moment and then talks about her self as ugly and undesirable. The psychologist interrupts her and asks Deb to use words that describe the physical nature of her body rather than in values like "undesirable." Deb has to think about this some more and then tells her that she sees her body as a desert, dry and hot and difficult to live in. With some more encouragement, she describes her genital area as raw and red and parched to a silvery white. The psychologist then asks Deb if she's looked at her body and in particular at her genitals. Deb is surprised by the question; why would she want to look at herself down there? She's tired of people looking at her down there. Brent had to look at her down there, and she just wants "down there" to go away. The psychologist suggests to Deb that she go home and get a mirror and look at herself.

Dr. Katz Explains

This is a very useful strategy. How we see ourselves sometimes influences how we feel and act. Deb states clearly that she feels undesirable and has an image of her genitals as red and raw at the same time as they are dry and fragile. Telling Brent this also can help him to understand why she feels so differently about herself than he thinks of her.

Take-Away Points

- If you've experienced treatment that has caused lasting physical effects, take a few minutes to put into words how you see your body in your mind. Even better, take some crayons and draw what you feel and think your body looks like. You may be surprised at the results.
- A psychologist or mental health practitioner can be very helpful in dealing with the emotional side of illness. In partnership with your physical care providers, he or she can really help with healing and recovery.

Love Hurts

The next time they try to have sex, Deb's once again in a lot of pain. Brent's afraid of hurting her and watches her face closely. As soon as he sees her grimace, he stops and tells her that he's not going to touch her again until she's sure that it won't hurt. Deb's not sure when that day will be. She calls her nurse practitioner and recounts what has happened over the last few months. The nurse practitioner asks her to come in again, and this time she examines Deb's genitalia. She tells Deb that, as she probably knows, she's really dry there and suggests a strategy to deal with this. She instructs Deb to buy a vaginal moisturizer from the drugstore and to use it three times a week to increase the moisture level of her vagina. She also talks to Deb about using a lubricant for sexual activity; Deb replies that sex is not going to happen unless the pain goes away. Finally, she tells Deb that if the vaginal moisturizer does not work, she's going to suggest that she use estrogen in the vagina to help to replenish the tissues.

Deb buys some vaginal moisturizer from the drugstore and follows the package directions. After about two weeks, she feels more comfortable, and it is certainly easier to use the dilators now. She had been using K-Y® Jelly (McNeil-PPC, Inc.) that she got from the cancer center. Deb and Brent try to have sex once again—this time it's Brent's birthday—and once again it really hurt, and they couldn't do anything. She feels so bad for him. He tries so hard not to let her see that he's frustrated, but she can see it.

Take-Away Point

- Your healthcare provider is not necessarily an expert in the different kinds of lubricants that are available. Try going to your local sex store, where staff will know the pros and cons of all their products. Or look online, where you can find an extensive range of companies that specialize in these items.

Dr. Katz Explains

There are different solutions for different situations. Replens® ('Lil Drug Store Products, Inc.) is a vaginal moisturizer that allows water to move into the vaginal walls. It is a gel that is inserted with an applicator into the vagina three times a week. It takes about two weeks for the effects to be felt. You can purchase this product at any drugstore without a prescription. It is not recommended for use during intercourse.

To make intercourse easier, a lubricant is the appropriate choice. Many lubricants are available, and some can be found at your local drugstore, whereas others are only available at sex stores or online. Two types of lubricants are most effective. Glycerin-based lubricants (e.g., Astroglide® [BioFilm, Inc.], K-Y Liquid) are very slick and stay this way for a long time, so they do not dry up during sexual activity. They may increase yeast in the vagina and may be a concern if you have frequent yeast infections. Silicone-based lubricants also are very effective but are more difficult to find and may have to be purchased online or in sex stores. Also available are water-based lubricants that do not contain glycerin (e.g., Liquid Silk® [Bodywise Ltd.]); these usually can be found online or in sex stores.

It's Getting Better All the Time

Deb calls the nurse practitioner the next day and tells her that perhaps she needs more than the Replens. The nurse practitioner prescribes estrogen tablets, which Deb receives the next week. They are small, and the instructions say to insert them once a day for two weeks and then twice a week. After 10 days, Deb notices a real change. She feels almost normal again and is happy that, at last, something has worked. The thought of sex still does not excite her, but she has a glimmer of hope that this might work.

Dr. Katz Explains

A local estrogen treatment, such as Deb was prescribed, will help the vaginal tissues to regain moisture from the inside. This is the best treatment for severe vaginal dryness. Estrogen comes in a number of different forms: cream, pills, and a ring that is placed in the vagina and remains there for 90 days, at which time it's replaced by a new one.

The Promise of a Happy Ending

That weekend, Deb snuggles up to Brent after dinner. They're sitting on the deck with a glass of wine, and she suggests that perhaps they can try again. Brent is cautious; the thought of her in pain again is almost too much for him, but she seems interested for the first time in months.

This time he is able to insert his penis into her vagina with only a little difficulty. He watches her closely, and while she does not seem excited, she's not in pain like before. He hurries to finish; after such a long time, this is easy to do. She seems happy that she had no pain, and even though she didn't really experience any satisfaction herself, it's enough for her to see Brent satisfied. It's a beginning.

CHAPTER 8

Multiple Losses

Will it ever be the way it was?

Being diagnosed with cancer can lead to many different feelings, including depression. This may last for months or years after treatment has ended. Being cured doesn't mean that your fears are gone, and some people suffer in silence without ever getting help.

Many effective treatments for depression are available, and most people will respond well to them. But some people also experience side effects from these medications. Depression often is treated with a group of medications called selective serotonin reuptake inhibitors (SSRIs). You may have taken these yourself or know someone who has taken them. But one of the most common side effects of these medications is sexual difficulties.

In this chapter, you will meet Rebecca and Don. Rebecca was successfully treated for skin cancer but finds herself depressed three years after. You will learn

- How depression can affect your sex life
- How treatment for depression can affect sexuality both negatively and positively.

Rebecca's Story

Rebecca and Don are both in their early 60s. Rebecca was successfully treated for malignant skin cancer three years ago. In her youth, she spent summers working as a lifeguard and even as an adult loved to spend time in the sun. Don noticed a mole on her back one night when they were undressing for bed.

Her family physician thought it looked suspicious and removed it under local anesthetic. The pathology report described it as a stage 0 malignant melanoma, and she was referred to a surgical oncologist, who performed a wide excision to ensure that there was no cancer left. Since then, she's been cancer free.

Dr. Katz Explains

Melanoma is a serious form of skin cancer that is associated with sun exposure. Rebecca has always spent time in the sun, and she was lucky that her husband noticed the mole and she was able to have prompt treatment. This cancer was caught at an early stage when removal of the cancerous lesion was the only treatment necessary.

Rebecca and Don both are retired and lead active lives. They live in a retirement community on the outskirts of a large city and enjoy golf, dancing, and travel. They never had children and have a strong relationship and a great sex life. But since her cancer, Rebecca is just different.

Being Different

Don can't really describe how she's different. She seems to do what she used to do, but she is somehow just not "there" when she does it. Her laughter is at times a little forced, and she no longer makes social arrangements spontaneously but rather waits for friends to call her or for Don to suggest they see their friends. She's lost weight but doesn't want to talk about it, and while she fills her plate at meals, Don has noticed that she pushes the food around rather than eating it.

Their sex life has suffered as well. Where once she was uninhibited and really enjoyed sex, she's now distant and appears to Don to be no longer interested in sex—and perhaps even him. Don doesn't know what to do; when he asks her what's wrong, she bristles and says that everything's fine. He's worried about her and is sure that things aren't fine.

Dr. Katz Explains

Everyone reacts differently to a diagnosis of cancer. Some people take it in stride, get through the treatment, and move on with their lives. Others find it more difficult regardless of the kind of cancer or the treatment. Rebecca was lucky in that her cancer was at an early stage when it was diagnosed, and yet she seems different three years afterward. There is no right or wrong way to respond to a cancer diagnosis; individual reactions are very different.

The situation can be very difficult for the partner of someone who has cancer. He or she may not be sure how to respond to changes in behavior. Don has noticed some significant changes in his wife; she is distant and is no longer the same social person she once was. Her appetite has decreased, and she is losing weight. She's also lost interest in sex, which bothers him. When he asks her if she's okay, he gets a negative response, and this may mean that he doesn't ask her again. It's not uncommon for the partner to feel like he's walking on eggshells in a situation like this.

Take-Away Points

- Don has noticed some changes that are concerning him. It's good to listen to your gut and respond to your observations of change in a partner.
- Even though you may tell your partner that everything's all right, it may not be so. Persistence is a good thing in a case like this.

Opening Up

Before Rebecca's annual follow-up appointment at the cancer center, Don suggests that they ask to see a counselor. Rebecca reacts with a hasty retort that perhaps *he* needs a counselor, but she's fine. Don breaks down; through his tears he asks her if she wants to divorce him. She's shocked; she wonders what brought this on. This is perhaps the second time in the 40 years of their marriage that she's seen him cry. The reality of this makes her sit down next to him and listen.

He tells her that from his point of view, she's acting like someone who's no longer interested in him or their marriage. Or she's having an affair. Hearing this, she starts to laugh but then realizes that he's serious, and she hurries to reassure him that neither is true. She tells him that she loves him very much, and even though she doesn't really understand what he's talking about, she wants to understand. And she agrees to see a counselor.

Take-Away Points

- Don't be afraid to expose your feelings to your partner. Sometimes it's necessary in order to make changes.
- Our partners may misunderstand our actions and misinterpret what is happening. That's what happens when people don't talk to each other.
- Eventually the truth will come out, even if it's in the midst of tears.

Dr. Katz Explains

Don is trying to reach out to Rebecca, but she can't see that until he does something quite out of character: he cries. This gets her attention. Don has to explain that, from his perspective, she is acting as if their marriage is over. This is hard to hear, especially when she knows that it isn't true. Often, it takes something like this to make us sit up and take notice of how our behavior is affecting someone else.

Asking for Help

At her appointment, Rebecca tells the nurse that she'd like to see a counselor. The nurse replies that she'll see if the social worker who works with the team is available. Don and Rebecca are surprised that it's happening so fast; they've not really formulated their questions or concerns. After Rebecca sees the oncologist, the nurse tells the couple that the social worker wants to introduce herself to them.

After five minutes, a smiling middle-aged woman pokes her head around the door. She introduces herself as Sandy and asks them if they could come in to see her later that week. They agree to an early morning appointment at the end of the week.

Friday soon arrives, and Rebecca and Don make their way to the cancer center. They've not talked much about this appointment, but the atmosphere between them has softened. The waiting room in the social work department is warm and inviting. Large plants grow in front of the windows, and there's a pile of magazines on a side table. The receptionist offers them coffee or tea, which they decline. Sandy comes out of her office a few minutes later. They follow her to her office, which is also filled with plants. They sit in comfortable chairs while she faces them from a short distance.

"Tell me why you're here," she says, and they both hesitate for an instant. And then Don starts to speak. He struggles to maintain his composure as he describes how afraid he's been about the state of their marriage. Rebecca doesn't make eye contact with him while he talks. She twists a button on her sweater and gazes into her lap. Sandy waits until Don is finished and then asks Rebecca how she sees the situation. Rebecca shrugs and appears to find difficulty speaking.

Dr. Katz Explains

Each member of a couple has his or her own understanding and interpretation of what is happening at any time in the relationship. Don sees the situation as a threat to their marriage. But his opinion is not the only opinion, and it's important to hear what Rebecca has to say. She is the one whose behavior has changed the dynamics of this relationship, and her thoughts are paramount. But it is difficult for her to express herself, and Don jumped in when they were asked why they were at the appointment. This is also not unusual; Don was just taking charge in Rebecca's silence.

Letting It All Out, Part 1

After a long silence in which Don looks imploringly at her and then at Sandy as if trying to coax either of them to speak first, Rebecca takes a deep breath and begins. She talks about feeling disconnected from everything. She doesn't look at Don as she describes feeling completely alone and lonely. Don looks as if he is going to interrupt her, but Sandy puts out her hand, and he closes his mouth. Rebecca continues to describe her feelings of isolation. She acknowledges that she's let things slide but that she's just so tired and after three years she wants to feel better.

Sandy asks her if she's sleeping well, and Rebecca admits that she wakes in the early hours, long before Don, and she lies in bed, willing herself to feel better and just get on with things. She looks at Don when she says that she has no appetite and gets irritated when she sees him watching her playing with her food at meals. Don blushes, and Rebecca manages a small smile that barely lifts the corners of her mouth.

At this point, Sandy gently suggests to Rebecca that perhaps she's depressed. Rebecca seems puzzled by this and tells Sandy that she's never been depressed a day in her life. Don starts to agree, but instead he asks Sandy why she thinks that. Sandy explains that Rebecca has some of the signs of depression—early waking, loss of appetite, loss of interest in social relationships, fatigue—and that this is common in people with cancer, no matter what type of cancer or how long since diagnosis. Rebecca seems upset by this and gets up and moves swiftly to the door. As she opens it, she looks back at Don, who glances briefly at Sandy and follows his wife.

Take-Away Points

- If you're feeling sad or your usual lifestyle is altered in any way, tell someone about it.
- Depression is very common and needs to be treated. There is no shame in asking for help for this.

Dr. Katz Explains

Rebecca is showing some of the classic signs of depression. She is waking early in the morning, has lost her appetite, no longer experiences pleasure in social events, and even avoids other people when she can. She is distant with her husband and finds it difficult to explain how she is feeling. And her response to the social worker also is not unusual; she is upset, and her response to others is unpredictable.

Depression is common in people who have cancer, and it's sometimes not given the attention it deserves. Rebecca's treatment was fairly straightforward—she had surgery to remove the mole on her back—and she has only had yearly follow-up appointments. Often, when treatment is more complex and there are more opportunities to interact with the healthcare team, someone will ask how the patient is feeling, and that is when depression is diagnosed. Some cancer centers ask patients to complete assessment forms at every visit that identify feelings of depression so that treatment can be initiated.

Letting It All Out, Part 2

They don't say much on the way home. Rebecca's embarrassed at her behavior, and Don doesn't know what to say. He thinks that Sandy may be right; Rebecca does seem to be depressed, and he can't figure out why her response was to leave the room suddenly. As soon as they walk in the door of their condo, Rebecca goes to the phone and calls Sandy to apologize. She asks if she can see Sandy alone, and they arrange an appointment for the following week. Don's pleased to hear this, and for the rest of the week he goes out of his way to give her space.

On Wednesday of the next week, Rebecca drives to the cancer center for her appointment with Sandy. She's nervous but at the same time eager to talk about some things that have been bothering her and that she can't talk to Don about. She feels guilty about this; for 40 years they've shared a life and their feelings. But things are different now; she's different and wants to find out how she can make things the same as they were before.

They start by talking about what happened at her last appointment. Sandy asks her why she reacted as she did when the subject of depression was raised. Sandy pauses for a moment and then tells Sandy that her mother had "emotional issues" and was sent to see a psychiatrist, who put her in the hospital for treatment. This happened when Rebecca was 16 years old, and her mother was gone for six months. The first time they went to see her, Rebecca hardly recognized the small woman in the bed. Her father bent over to kiss her on the cheek, and she pulled away with a wild look in her eyes. Rebecca was terrified—who was this woman and why did her father try to kiss her?—and pulled her younger brother out of the room with her. They waited outside in the hallway until their father came out of the room. She could tell he was angry, but who was he angry with? Months later her mother returned home to her family; she was thin and pale and was never the same as Rebecca remembered.

Dr. Katz Explains

Our responses are not always rational or measured. Rebecca has some deep-rooted memories of a difficult time in her life, and this came rushing to the surface when Sandy mentioned depression. Rebecca recognizes that she's not dealing with things very well. She admits that she's hiding things from Don and can't share her feelings with him for the first time in their marriage. She also wants their life to be the same as it was before. This may not be possible because people change in response to what has happened to them.

> ### Take-Away Points
>
> - Your response to a situation may be influenced by experiences from your past. Even if you don't really want to think about what happened long ago, it may help you to understand why you're acting in a certain way now.
> - People change in response to illness, especially a life-threatening illness like cancer.
> - Things may not be the same as they were before; it's possible that they may be better.

Suggesting a Solution

Sandy listened intently to Rebecca's story, nodding slightly as Rebecca disclosed her feelings and fears buried deep in the memories. Sandy tells her that it's now easy to see why Rebecca might be upset to think that she's depressed. She thinks that Rebecca might need an antidepressant and asks Rebecca if she has strong feelings about those medications. Rebecca replies that she doesn't have strong feelings for or against them and has seen a friend's mood improve while on one. But she'd prefer not to go on one yet and asks if she can just wait and see how things go. Sandy suggests that she continue to see Rebecca and Don to work with them on any issues that they want to address. Rebecca feels a big weight lifted off her shoulders and agrees to another appointment in two weeks.

Dr. Katz Explains

Many people are reluctant to try medication for the treatment of depression. They think that they should be able to get over it and get better by themselves. This can work for some people, and a form of talk therapy has been shown to be effective, even as effective as medication.

The "S" Word

Don's pleased that Rebecca has agreed to continue with counseling. He finds that over time, her mood seems to be lighter. At their next appointment with

Sandy, he asks the social worker if it's normal this far from treatment for Rebecca to be so disinterested in sex. Rebecca gasps when he says this. They've not talked about this at all, and she feels betrayed that he's brought this up without talking to her first. Sandy asks a few questions and then tells them that they really should see the sexuality counselor who works at the cancer center. At this point Rebecca just wants to get out of Sandy's office, so she agrees to have Sandy talk to whoever this sexuality counselor is. Once again they drive home in silence, but this time, it's an angry silence.

Dr. Katz Explains

Rebecca feels ambushed by Don raising the topic of sex with Sandy without telling her that he's going to do it. She's right; he really should have talked to her first. But sometimes people do things out of desperation and don't think about what's right and what's not.

Take-Away Point

- Talk to your partner if you're going to a medical or support appointment. Share your plan about what you want to talk about.

It Takes Two to Tango

Don tries to explain to Rebecca why he did this; she tells him that she needs to get over his betrayal of her and that it's going to take some time. He apologizes and asks her just to listen to him, but she's too angry. Two days later she's cooled off a bit, and after dinner she tells him she's ready to listen. He once again apologizes and describes how lonely he feels and how much he misses their old life, which now seems like a far-away dream. She's moved by his words and admits that she, too, remembers what they had as a dream because what she's experiencing now is a nightmare. They both find themselves in tears, and she promises him that she'll see the sexuality counselor and will find a way to make things better. Don tells her that he's going to go to all her appointments with her unless she or the healthcare provider specifically requests that he not be there. She agrees and, for the first time in a long while, smiles with her mouth, her eyes, and her heart.

Dr. Katz Explains

It always helps to talk things through. Both partners are upset about the same things, and instead of fighting about them they'd do much better to share their feelings with each other. Rebecca's willingness to see the sexuality counselor indicates to him that she's as bothered by this as he is. His intention to go to all her appointments with her shows his commitment to their relationship.

Talking About It

The next morning, there's a call from the sexuality counselor at the cancer center. Rebecca agrees to meet with her the following week and asks if she should bring her spouse with her. The answer is "yes," and she tells Don that he's welcome to go along with her. A week later, they make the journey to the cancer center. The sexuality counselor, Gail, is a young woman with black hair and a big smile. She immediately puts both of them at ease with her warm welcome and casual but professional manner. Perhaps it won't be that bad.

Gail asks the couple a lot of questions. Don answers some, but mostly Rebecca talks. She describes being totally disinterested in sex for the last two years and admits that she really misses it and acknowledges that something has changed between her and Don as a result. She also admits to feeling really down and thinks that sex, or the lack of it, has something to do with it. This time it is Gail who gently suggests that Rebecca may be depressed. The couple agrees, and Rebecca quickly states that she doesn't want to see a psychiatrist. Gail tells Rebecca that her family physician is quite capable of dealing with this and suggests that Rebecca make an appointment to see him and describe how she's feeling. She suggests a follow-up appointment with her after she's seen her family physician.

Dr. Katz Explains

Rebecca is finally ready to accept some help. This time when the sexuality counselor suggests that she is depressed, she is ready to accept that. She realizes that there *is* a connection between the way she is feeling and her lack of interest in sex. But she is still reluctant to see a psychiatrist.

Take-Away Points

- We all have different reasons for getting help. There are no right or wrong reasons; the important thing is to get the help.
- Usually, different options are available for getting the help you need. Be open to them.

On the Road to Wellness

Rebecca hasn't seen her family physician for a while, but she likes him. She calls his clinic and is pleased to hear that there's an opening early the next week. Don once again accompanies her to this appointment and is impressed with the assessment that Dr. Carter does. They walk out of the clinic with a prescription for an antidepressant. Rebecca seems to think this is the same medication that her friend took. She takes the first one that night and within three weeks seems much brighter. Don can notice the difference, too, and once again there is laughter in their house.

Dr. Katz Explains

With a few questions as part of an assessment, most competent practitioners can diagnose depression. Rebecca has some of the classic signs, and medication usually will help. And many people do start to feel better within three or four weeks of starting the antidepressant medication.

More Talk

They see the sexuality counselor, Gail, a few weeks after their first appointment. Rebecca was already feeling better, and they talk about the changes in their relationship. Gail listens to their descriptions, nodding occasionally but mostly just letting them talk to each other. Don admits that for him, Rebecca's enjoyment of sex was a sign that she loved him and that he'd been surprised at his response when things weren't going well. He didn't think after all the time they'd been married that he'd be so insecure. Rebecca doesn't say much in response to this other than that she loves him and is sorry that he felt like this. The hour-long appointment is soon over, and they make plans to meet again in two weeks.

Dr. Katz Explains

Even after many years of marriage, it's still possible to feel insecure when things change. Don had taken Rebecca's enjoyment of sex to mean something about her feelings for him. This was his interpretation, and it's no wonder that when sex was no longer something they shared, he might be unsure of her feelings for him. Once again, this isn't necessarily rational but is just part of the way we are as human beings.

A Problem Arises

At their next appointment with Gail, Don and Rebecca seem much closer. Rebecca's depression has lifted, and she is once again doing all the things she enjoyed. There is just one problem: although they've started having sex again, Rebecca isn't enjoying it as much. Rebecca describes being interested in sex again, which is a huge relief, but for the first time in her life is unable to have an orgasm. Don admits that this is making him feel bad; he'd always prided himself on satisfying his partner, and this was frustrating for him. Once or twice he'd even lost his erection while they were making love, and he is now worried that this would happen every time.

Gail explains that the kind of antidepressant that Rebecca is taking has some sexual side effects, including the effect she was seeing on her ability to have an orgasm. The question is what Rebecca and Don want to do about it. They have some choices: stay on the medication and find a way to deal with the sexual changes, change to another medication, or try to find a way of treating the lack of orgasms. Don and Rebecca seem deflated; just when she is feeling better mentally, this had to happen.

Dr. Katz Explains

A side effect of this class of antidepressants, the SSRIs, is difficulty having an orgasm. Women who were previously easily orgasmic may find that they really struggle to have an orgasm while on these medications. This side effect is very common, occurring in 20%–70% of people taking them and leading to many people stopping the medication in the first few months. This may then lead to recurrence of the depression.

Rebecca experienced absent orgasm as a side effect, but other side effects include lack of interest in sex, decreased genital sensitivity and lubrication, pain with intercourse, and decrease in sexual activity and sexual satisfaction. Switching to another antidepressant may help, but this usually involves a period between stopping the one medication and starting the other one; signs of depression may return in this time period.

A recent study showed that premenopausal women who experience sexual side effects of antidepressants can be treated effectively with sildenafil, one of the medications used to treat erectile dysfunction in men. This trial only involved women who were not past menopause, and there is no evidence that this would be effective for someone like Rebecca, who is older than the women in the study.

Take-Away Points

- It's important to tell the healthcare provider who prescribed the medication for you if you notice any sexual changes.
- Your healthcare provider may not tell you that these changes are possible, so be prepared to advocate for yourself.
- You may have to weigh the different options. Think about what is most important for you, and then make your decision.

Working Out the Kinks

Rebecca tells Gail that she really doesn't want to get depressed again. She's feeling so much better, and she'd rather try another medication than quit completely. Gail supports her in this decision, and Don looks really relieved. Rebecca makes a follow-up appointment with her family physician, as well as another appointment with Gail for later that month. Gail encourages the couple to keep touching and talking. Don has a naughty grin on his face as they leave; he's almost gotten the old Rebecca back, and he's going to do everything to prevent her from going away again.

Rebecca sees Dr. Carter early the next week. She tells him that although she's feeling better, she's having problems in her sex life and wants to do something about it. Dr. Carter checks something in a large book on his desk and writes her a prescription for another antidepressant. This one is called bupropion, and he tells her that this has a better sexual side effect profile than the other medications in this class. Rebecca can't help wondering why he didn't prescribe that for her in the first place.

Dr. Katz Explains

Unfortunately, sex is not a topic that is freely discussed, even in the doctor's office. This is not something that most doctors or nurse practitioners think about when prescribing medications. Luckily there is an alternative for the treatment of depression that may help, and this is what Dr. Carter has prescribed for Rebecca.

It's Getting Better All the Time

Rebecca starts taking the new medication and two weeks later is a little surprised when she feels something she has not felt for a while. The sight of Don cutting the grass causes her to feel a tingly sensation she'd almost forgotten she could feel. She calls him in from outside, and even though he's sweaty and covered in tiny pieces of grass, she pulls him toward her and gives him a long, passionate kiss. Don's very surprised but in the nicest way. In response to her kiss, he picks her up in his arms and carries her to the bedroom. He takes a quick shower and returns to the bedroom dripping wet. They make love hurriedly, and they're both surprised at her response. She's not sure if this orgasm is so much better because it's been a while since she had one, but they're both really pleased that things are working again.

Dr. Katz Explains

Bupropion is an antidepressant that is known to actually enhance sexual functioning, unlike the others, which seem to diminish sexual interest and response. The more positive side effects of this particular drug include increased libido, increased genital arousal, enhanced ability to have an orgasm, and orgasms that are more intense than before.

A Happy Ending

The next time Rebecca and Don see Gail, they are holding hands in the waiting room. They report that the last few weeks have been the best of their life together. Rebecca is energetic and happy again. Their social life has improved, and they have a calendar full of golf games and outings with their friends. And Don can't help blurting out that he's got a whole new confidence in his ability to please Rebecca. His smile when he says this lights up the room. The couple express their gratitude to Gail for helping them through this sticky patch and tell her that they don't need to see her again. Things are great once again, and besides, they just don't have the time to spend on appointments anymore.

CHAPTER 9

Communication

I have something to tell you.

Communication about sex often is difficult in the face of life-threatening illness. The challenges for the single cancer survivor are perhaps even more significant. When do you tell a new sexual partner that you have lost a breast or part of your colon, that you can't have children, or that you've been treated for cancer?

In this chapter, you'll meet Angela, who's 31 years old and has been treated for Hodgkin lymphoma. She's single and finds it difficult to know when to tell a prospective partner that she had cancer. She's had a relationship fail and is very fearful about disclosure and ruining things.

In this chapter, you'll learn

- How to tell someone that you've had cancer
- When to tell a potential partner that you've had cancer.

Angela's Story

Angela lives in a large city in California. She moved there with her boyfriend about five years ago and was just starting to make friends. Everything was going well: She'd found a great job at a local TV station where she was a production assistant, and she loved the weather after spending most of her life in Minnesota. She came down with what she thought was the flu about three years after moving there. She didn't think much about it, but she didn't get

109

better and after six weeks, still felt tired and had no appetite. One day in the shower, she felt a lump in her neck. She thought this was part of the flu, but her boyfriend suggested she see her doctor because she'd been sick for a long time and was not getting better.

Bad News

She was shocked when her family physician sent her for a biopsy of the lump and learned it was Hodgkin lymphoma. Within two weeks, she began chemotherapy treatment. She had a difficult time with this and felt ill almost all the time. Her boyfriend took great care of her when he was around; he'd joined a new IT company and traveled a lot, so he was only there two days a week. But she got through it, and when her treatment was done she was 25 pounds thinner, bald, and very, very tired. But she was in remission.

She had to quit her job soon after she started chemotherapy. Because she had not been there long and the job had limited benefits, her sick time ran out quickly. Tim, her boyfriend, had a good job and was paying the rent on their small apartment. It took her three months to start feeling better after the chemo. Most days she sat on the balcony, watching the traffic go by. If she felt okay, she'd go to the store and buy something to eat, but she mostly just waited for Tim to come back from his travels.

Bad News Again

Almost one year to the day of her diagnosis, she went to the oncologist for her regular appointment. She was feeling better, but she was still really tired all the time. She had the usual blood tests and went home to wait for Tim to come back. She didn't expect the phone call from the oncologist, which came later that afternoon. Her blood tests were abnormal: the cancer was back.

Dr. Katz Explains

Some people don't stay in remission, and further treatment is necessary. This is heartbreaking after going through chemotherapy once. It's as if once you know what treatment is going to be like, it's even harder than the first time.

Coping, but Barely

For the next few weeks, she felt like she was walking in a fog. She had multiple visits to the oncologist, she was asked to make a lot of decisions about what would happen next, and she had to do it all alone. Tim was away doing a big project, and even though he said he was sorry he wasn't there, Angela had a sneaking suspicion that part of him was really glad to be away and not involved in everything. But she was too scared and tired to think about that a lot. The nurses at the cancer center were wonderful, and one of her neighbors kept an eye on her.

Dr. Katz Explains

Cancer treatment is all about making decisions, sometimes even when you're not sure exactly what's happening. Your healthcare providers can help and guide you, but ultimately you have to decide what comes next. This can be very difficult when you don't have someone with whom to discuss it. Even though you're the only one who'll have to go through the treatment, having supportive people around you can really help.

A Battle and Then More Bad News

After many visits to the oncologist, the treatment team recommended that she receive a bone marrow transplant. First they took out some of her bone marrow. Then she was admitted to the hospital, where she had massive doses of chemotherapy to kill off her remaining bone marrow. When this was over, her frozen cells were given back to her. For a number of weeks, she was in the hospital in isolation. She only saw the staff's eyes over their masks as they were completely covered in gowns, gloves, caps, and masks to prevent her from getting an infection. She felt really sick through all of this. But the worst part was that she hardly heard from Tim. When she first went into the hospital, he sent her e-mails every day, but soon these slowed down, and eventually she didn't hear from him for days in a row. By the time she was ready to go home, she knew the relationship was over. When she got to the apartment, his stuff was gone; there was a note saying he was sorry, but he just couldn't handle it anymore. He'd moved out but had paid the rent for the next six months.

Dr. Katz Explains

A bone marrow transplant is difficult to get through. For weeks, you're kept in isolation to avoid any chance of infection while your body's defenses are absent. And watching a relationship die during this time is especially difficult. Not everyone behaves in an ethical manner when someone else is sick. Relationships do come to an end. A health crisis such as this may be just too much for some people to cope with, and they're not honorable or kind and they leave.

Moving On

Over the next three months, Angela slowly recovered. Her hair started to grow back, and she gained some strength. She started looking for a new apartment; the one she shared with Tim was too big for her, and the memories weren't doing her any good. She found a small apartment in a quiet back street just three blocks from the ocean. She couldn't believe her luck. To be this close to the water was a dream come true for a young woman from Minnesota. She'd found the apartment through one of the nurses at the cancer center. Nina was about the same age as Angela and had been really supportive when she learned Angela's cancer had come back. In fact, Nina lived in the same apartment block, and they bumped into each other at the mailboxes once or twice a week.

The weeks and months flew by. Angela grew stronger every day and was soon thinking about going back to work but first had to find a job. She thought about calling the TV station where she worked when she first moved here but was nervous that they'd not want to take her on after she'd gotten sick while working there. One day she came home from a walk (she'd started walking along a path by the beach every morning) and the message light was flashing on her answering machine. It was the TV station. Her former manager wanted to know if she was ready to come back to her old job. Angela was stunned and stood on her tiny balcony with tears pouring down her face. This was just too good to be true. It was almost as if someone had been reading her thoughts.

She started work two weeks later. The crew in the production department all seemed pleased to see her. Her hair was shorter than it was when she was last there; it had grown out curly, and she hadn't bothered putting in highlights so it was much darker. No one said anything about her hair, and everyone acted as if all was normal and nothing had happened in the intervening 18 months. Angela was a little surprised that nothing was said about her hair, her absence, or anything related to her cancer, but she was soon back in the swing of things, and work was really busy.

Dr. Katz Explains

Sometimes people really don't know what to say and so say nothing. They may be afraid of saying the wrong thing or of the kind of response they may get. This can be hurtful; it's as if everything you've gone through didn't happen.

Take-Away Points

- If you want to talk about anything—your hair, what it was like having treatment—just go ahead and speak up.
- People will take their lead from you; if you talk about it, they'll ask questions if they want to.
- Sometimes using humor can really help to break the ice. A well-timed joke may open the door to making others feel more comfortable asking you how you are.

Getting Back in the Swing of Things

Angela loved being back at work. Even though the long days were really tiring, she felt energized when she got into work in the mornings. There were some new people working with her, and one, in particular, was really interesting. His name was Joe, and he worked in the graphics end of things. They'd talked in the lunchroom, and she'd definitely gotten signals that he might be interested in her.

On Thursday at the end of the day, a group of her coworkers all left at the same time. They talked in the elevator about going out for a drink, and Angela agreed to join them. On their way out of the building they bumped into Joe, who was getting his bike off the bike rack. One of the men invited him along, and she noticed him glance over in her direction. She felt her heart flutter just a little bit and ran her hand through her hair, making sure it wasn't standing up.

They ended up on the patio of a bar about three blocks from the TV station. It was a warm evening, and the sky was purple and orange as the sun went down. Suddenly Joe was standing next to her, and they smiled shyly at one another. They made small talk—Where do you live? Where do you come from?—and soon they were sitting by themselves, slightly away from the group. The evening sped by, and with a start she realized it was almost midnight and tomorrow was going to be even busier than today. Joe offered to walk back to the station with her to pick up her car and his bike. When they got back to the station, he asked her to have dinner with him on Saturday night. She was glad it was dark because she could feel her face turning red. She agreed and gave him her address and drove away, her hands shaking slightly on the steering wheel.

The next day was really busy at work, and she didn't see him before she left for the weekend. She was really excited; this was her first date since Tim left, and she was a little scared, too. She spent most of Saturday pacing her apartment. She went for a walk, and on her way back, she saw Nina, the nurse from the cancer center. They greeted each other and fell into an easy conversation. Nina told her that she looked great, and she told Nina that she had a date that night. They spent 30 minutes talking and laughing in the front hall of the apartment block and then parted ways. Nina went up the stairs to her apartment and Angela to hers, where she continued to pace, watching the clock every few minutes.

The First Date

At five minutes before seven o'clock her buzzer sounded; it was Joe, and he was early. She tried to take her time going down the stairs, but she couldn't help herself and within seconds was at the door. His hair was still wet from the shower, and he was wearing a bright cotton shirt with colorful fishes all over it. He looked different from how he looked at work, but the smile was the same. He'd borrowed his brother's car for the evening, and they took off for a fish place about 30 minutes away.

They talked easily on the way to the restaurant, mostly about work. As the night went on, they talked about their childhoods and found lots in common. Again, the evening sped by, and she hardly noticed the food or the wine. She really liked him; he had a good sense of humor, and they talked easily about all sorts of things. Before she knew it, the meal was over and she was shocked to look at her watch and see that it was past 11 pm. They got up to leave, and soon they were in the car and then at her apartment. He kissed her on the cheek at the door and left with a smile and a wave. And then it hit her: She didn't talk about her cancer at all. She didn't even think about it for a minute on the date, but now she's not sure what to do about it. She needed to tell him, but she hadn't, and how was she going to do it now?

Dr. Katz Explains

After months of feeling sick, Angela is feeling back to normal and is ready to date. This is a good sign of her recovery and not just from the bone marrow transplant but also from her breakup with Tim. But dating again or the start of a new relationship leads to the important topic of when to tell someone that you've had cancer.

What to Do?

She thought about this a lot the next day. When should she tell him? Maybe he already knew. Perhaps someone at work had told him. Maybe she won't date him again, and does he need to know? Once again she found herself pacing her apartment. But she had an idea, and before she could change her mind, she went down the stairs and knocked on Nina's door. She's a nurse and works at the cancer center, and she seemed really friendly when they saw each other in the hallway. Angela repeated these thoughts as she approached Nina's door and knocked tentatively.

Nina answered the door; she was wrapped in a towel, and her hair was dripping all over the floor. They both apologized at the same time and started to laugh. She asked Angela to wait a few minutes and then reappeared in a fluffy robe (Angela has one just like it) and offered to make some tea. Soon they were chatting away like old friends. But Angela came here with a purpose, and she asked Nina how to handle telling Joe about her cancer.

Nina was thoughtful for a moment and then told her that she wasn't sure but said that some people seem to wait a while until the relationship looks like it's going somewhere. That's what Angela thought, and they talked for a few more minutes and Angela left.

- Trust your instincts, and tell when you think the time is right.
- There's no right or wrong way to do this. Just get the words out and then wait for the other person to say something or ask a question.
- You don't have to give all the details at once. Start simply and see where things go.

Dr. Katz Explains

There's no perfect time to tell someone that you've had cancer. But at some point, you do need to share this information. It's probably better to do this when it looks like a relationship is developing. This can be scary; rejection is always a possibility that can hurt, especially if this is the first time you've been interested in someone since treatment. So the first date is probably not the time to tell, but the second or third date may be just right.

After the Date

The next day at work she saw Joe going into his office, and they waved at each other. She was really nervous and hoped that she didn't turn red. Some of her coworkers knew about her date, and they were eager to hear all the details. They needed to be careful, though, as Joe could have appeared at any minute, so they left the studio for a few minutes at lunch time and walked to a coffee shop nearby. Angela was pleased that she wouldn't have to see Joe in the lunchroom, but she was also a little sad because part of her really wanted to see him again and talk to him.

Just before she left for the day, she was startled to see Joe standing at her desk, right behind her. She felt her face turn red, but he didn't seem to notice. He asked her if she'd like to go for a bike ride after work the next day. Angela was embarrassed to admit that she didn't own a bike, but Joe told her that his roommate has one that she could borrow. Once again, her heart was racing, but part of the reason was that she knew she was going to have to tell him. And she needed to do it soon.

Date Number 2

The next day after work, they met at the bike rack. She hoped he had a helmet for her, and she found him waiting there with everything she needed.

He even brought a bottle of water for her and a small towel. They rode toward the beach taking side roads and being really careful of the traffic. He took it slow and made sure she was keeping up with him. Soon they reached the beach and chained the bikes to a lamppost outside an ice cream store. They sat at a table on the patio and ate their ice cream. They had a lot to talk about once again, and the time flew. They rode back to the TV studio, and as she was getting back into her car, she found the words flowing out of her mouth. "I have something to tell you . . ."

Dr. Katz Explains

Angela is starting to have feelings for Joe and realizes that she needs to be honest with him if there's going to be anything between them. And as sometimes happens, without much planning the words just come out.

Take-Away Points

- Sometimes the perfect situation presents itself and the words come right out.
- Don't overthink it. Just start somewhere.
- It's better to know the truth—will he run or will he stay—than to be constantly afraid of what his reaction may be.

Getting It All Out

Her heart was beating in her throat as she said the words: "I have something to tell you. I had cancer. I also had a bone marrow transplant. I'm okay now. At least I think I am. I've been cancer-free for nine months now. I don't know what else to tell you . . ." At this point she remembered to take a breath. Her heart was beating so loudly that she could hear it in her ears. She couldn't even look at him because she was so scared about what she might see on his face. She just stood there with the car door open and the alarm dinging. After what seemed like forever but was really only seconds, Joe put his hand under her chin and raised her face to look at him. He was not smiling but his face was kind, and he told her that his sister had the same cancer when she was 35 years old. And she's fine now. And he's fine with knowing. And he's glad that she told him. And would she go out with him again on the weekend? It was going to be all right.

CHAPTER 10

Lesbians With Cancer

How do you know how I feel?

Lesbians sometimes are marginalized in their experience of cancer. There are some unique factors affecting lesbians' interactions in the healthcare system. Do you need to disclose your sexual orientation to get good medical care? Do people really need to know, and how does knowing or not knowing make a difference?

In this chapter, you'll hear how Noreen and her partner of 20 years successfully negotiated the cancer journey but not without some challenges along the way. Noreen, who is 45 years old, was diagnosed with osteosarcoma at the age of 25 and has a below-the-knee amputation. Her partner, Jen, is diagnosed with breast cancer 20 years later and has some problems coping within the healthcare system even though she is a nurse.

In this chapter, you'll learn
- What lesbians may experience in the healthcare system
- The pros and cons of disclosing your sexual orientation to your healthcare providers.

Noreen's Story

Noreen and Jen, a couple in their 40s, live in a small house in Seattle. They have two cats and a dog, and both women teach at a college that borders on their back fence. Noreen met Jen 20 years ago when she was hospitalized for a below-the-knee amputation of her right leg; she'd been diagnosed with osteosarcoma after she noticed a painful bump above her ankle that she thought was a sports injury. When it did not resolve, she saw a doctor; within two weeks she had the surgery, and her life changed forever.

During her hospital stay, Noreen was cared for by a woman named Jen who was about the same age and who had a great smile and a bubbly personality. Jen was a nurse who had recently moved to Seattle, and the two women instantly were attracted to each other. They were careful to hide this from each other and the rest of the world; nurses are not supposed to form relationships with patients. But the attraction was there, and after Noreen went home, she thought about "her" nurse often as she recuperated. Jen thought about "her" patient, too.

Six months later, they bumped into each other at a farmers' market. They literally bumped into each other; Noreen still was not adept on her crutches. She was trying to maneuver her way between the stalls at the market when she stumbled and bumped into someone behind her: Jen! The two women smiled at each other and started to talk. Soon they were sitting under a tree, and then the conversation moved to a nearby restaurant. Twenty years later, the conversation continues. They moved in together three months after they met again and have made a home and a life together. They now both teach at a community college; Jen teaches in the nursing department and Noreen in the geography department.

After 20 years, Noreen doesn't think about cancer much at all. The first few years after the diagnosis and surgery were difficult as she learned to use a prosthetic leg. She constantly was on alert for any sign that the cancer was back. But over time, the fears grew smaller and quieter and now are almost gone. Last year, Jen heard that the oncologist who treated Noreen had died; it was almost as if that was the last connection to her cancer.

Dr. Katz Explains

Time does pass, and the acuity of the cancer experience fades with the years. In the first years after cancer, every cough or sniff, slight ache or pain, brings the thought "Is the cancer back?" But when the cough is just a cough and the sniff is just a sniff, some confidence begins to build that not everything is a potential sign of recurrence.

The Normalcy of Couples

Noreen and Jen are, for the most part, very happy together. Jen's a neat freak, and Noreen's attitude toward housekeeping is a source of irritation to her. Noreen leaves papers, journals, magazines, and books everywhere. Jen's constantly picking them up and putting them in neat piles in their home office. Then Noreen gets mad because she can't find them and has no idea of where she was in her reading. But other than that, they get along just fine. They've made a life together, they have a close circle of friends, mostly teachers at the community college, and they love to travel in the summer and over the winter break.

This summer, two of their closest friends were getting married in California. Since that state allowed same-sex marriages in 2008, thousands of gay and lesbian couples have gotten married there. And Bobbie and Sue were doing it, too. About 100 people traveled to San Francisco for the wedding. The ceremony took place at a small hotel overlooking the ocean, and the party that night went on until the sun came up. The party guests staggered to their rooms after a dawn breakfast of scrambled eggs and smoked salmon.

Noreen and Jen were too wired to sleep. Seeing their dear friends get married had been so great, and once again they wondered if they should do it, too. They lay in bed talking about it, and Noreen idly stroked Jen's right breast as they dreamed out loud about what their wedding might be like. Suddenly Noreen stopped with her hand flat against her partner's breast. Jen kept on talking, not noticing the look on Noreen's face. Noreen couldn't move, and her hand felt like it was on fire but ice cold at the same time. She wanted to tell Jen to stop talking and feel what she's feeling, but she knew that once she said something, life would never be the same.

After a few moments, Jen noticed that Noreen was really quiet. She hardly noticed that her partner's hand was still on her breast. "Noreen, honey, what's the matter?" she asked. Noreen just sat there, with tears in her eyes, not daring to say the words. But Jen persisted and softly, so softly Noreen replied: "Jen, there's a lump in your breast. I felt it. Right here." Jen leaped off the bed and across the room to the lovely bathroom that just yesterday seemed palatial to them. "It can't be. I had a mammogram three months ago!" She slammed the bathroom door, and the room filled with a terrible silence. Noreen wanted to go in there with her but knew better. So she sat on the bed, not moving, just waiting.

After about 15 minutes Jen appeared in the doorway. Her jaw was clenched, and there were tears in her eyes. "I'm sorry. You're right. It's there. But why? And how?" Noreen had no answers to these questions. She went over and took Jen in her arms. She just held her for a long time as the room brightened in the morning sun. "Let's go home," she said, and wordlessly the couple packed their bags and prepared to travel back to Seattle and what lay ahead.

Dr. Katz Explains

A woman often discovers a breast lump in the shower, or her partner discovers it during sex. Despite regular mammograms, a breast lump may appear and the woman suddenly feels it—even in women who do regular breast self-exams.

Some people suggest that breast self-examination does more harm than good. Some women will find lumps, and this causes a great deal of anxiety and invasive tests such as biopsies that ultimately may be unnecessary. But tell that to a woman who found a lump while doing her monthly self-exam and was diagnosed with early breast cancer. To her, the self-exam was life-saving.

Facing the Truth

Jen saw her family physician within days of getting back to Seattle. She had an ultrasound and was sent to a surgeon who did a biopsy. And Jen heard the words that she was dreading: "It's cancer. But it's early. You have choices. Let's talk about them." The surgeon talked, and Jen sat there, not really listening and not hearing much. She hadn't included Noreen in any of these appointments even though if you asked her why, she didn't have a good reason. She just felt this was something she had to get through. After all, she was a nurse, and none of this was new to her.

She went for a long walk after this appointment and thought about things. She had a choice between lumpectomy and mastectomy, and the choice seemed clear to her. She wanted to save her breast, so she would have the lumpectomy followed by radiation.

Later that afternoon, she called the surgeon's office and scheduled the surgery and then called the head of the nursing department at the community college and told her that she needed a couple of weeks off. She did all this before Noreen came home. After dinner, which was eaten in silence, Jen laid it all out for Noreen. It was a cold and seemingly dispassionate recital of days and dates and times. Jen's jaw was clenched and her eyes steely as she talked about being off work for a few weeks and then seeing how the radiation went. Noreen sat there, dumbfounded. How had it come to this? Why was she only finding out about this now? Why had Jen cut her out like this?

Dr. Katz Explains

It's hard to anticipate how someone is going to react to a cancer diagnosis. Jen has withdrawn and dealt with everything by herself. Noreen could have been a real help and support for her—after all, she had cancer herself 20 years ago—but perhaps this is why Jen has cut her out. Each of us has to go through it in our own way. Even if it's not the best way.

Take-Away Points

- Get support where you want and from whom you want.
- Remember that sharing this burden can help to lighten the load; you don't have to do it alone.
- Even if you have a medical background, this time you're the patient, and it's different when it's happening to you.

Getting It Over and Done With

Jen had the surgery on a Monday morning. Even though she'd opted for removal of the lump only, she still had to undergo a general anesthetic. The surgeon also did something called a sentinel node biopsy, where dye is injected to see which lymph nodes take up the dye, and these are then removed. She woke up in the recovery room, and the first thing she saw was Noreen's face, naked under the bright lights and lined with worry. She smiled at her and reached for her hand. Perhaps the healing might begin right then.

Jen went home later that day with Noreen fussing over her. They were both tired and went to bed early. They still had not talked much, but there seemed to be a lessening of the tension between them. For the first time since they came back from San Francisco, Noreen slept through the night.

The next morning over breakfast the two women talked. Jen went first and started by apologizing for her behavior of the previous weeks. Noreen talked about her pain at being excluded at this important time. Jen had no real explanation and apologized again. But she was firm in her decision to do the rest alone; what was Noreen going to do anyway? She had to have radiation every day for five weeks. It was just a matter of showing up and getting it done. She could manage alone.

When It Starts to Hurt

Three weeks into her radiation therapy, Jen noticed that the skin over her right breast was very red and also painful. She talked to the radiation therapist, who suggested that she use cornstarch over the area. Over the next few days, it got worse, and Jen tried not to complain, but she was really bothered by this. Noreen tried to be supportive but was still smarting from being left out and found it difficult to be good-natured all the time.

Jen spoke to the radiation therapist again. She told her the cornstarch was not helping and now she had open blisters on the skin of her breast. The therapist, a young woman, told her to be sure to not let her husband touch that breast. Jen opened her mouth to correct her but closed it again. Why did she have to explain that she didn't have a husband but rather a . . . how would she describe Noreen? Her partner? Her lover? Both sounded wrong to her, but she just didn't feel like going into all that now, so she just shut her mouth.

Take-Away Points
• Not telling your health-care providers about your sexual orientation hides a part of you.
• This may affect whether the care you receive reflects the whole you because if a piece is missing—such as who your partner is—the care you receive may not be holistic.

Dr. Katz Explains

It's quite common to experience radiation damage to the skin over the area where the radiation is given. There are things you can do to prevent the burns, but inevitably there will be some damage. The radiation therapists will advise you on how to limit the damage and how to treat any that does occur.

The issue of disclosure of sexual orientation is more difficult to deal with. Many gays and lesbians do tell their healthcare providers that they are in a same-sex relationship and don't wait for an experience like this one, where the therapist has assumed that Jen has a husband. Like many other things in the cancer journey, there is no right or wrong way to go about disclosing sexual orientation or partner status to healthcare providers.

Whose Cancer Is This, Anyway?

Jen was exhausted by the time she had finished the course of treatment. She was buoyed by the news that the cancer had not spread. She had to have chemotherapy, however, and she faced that challenge with her usual stoicism. Noreen wanted to come with her to her appointment with the oncologist to discuss the chemotherapy, but Jen once again refused. She was a nurse. She knew about this, and, anyway, it was close to exam time at the college, and Noreen was really busy. Something that she couldn't say but really wanted to was that she was the one with cancer; Noreen's experience 20 years ago didn't matter anymore. But she didn't say it and went alone to this appointment, too.

Don't Ask, Don't Tell

Seeing the oncologist meant going through the whole family history and personal history again with the nurse who worked there. Jen was getting really sick of telling the same story over and over again but knew why the nurses had to ask the same questions. It was still irritating, however. When she was filling out the demographic form, she left out the part where it asked about marital status. She wasn't married or divorced or widowed. And she wasn't single. There wasn't a square for what she was, so she just left it out.

The nurse was kind and cheerful, just what Jen didn't need. She was tense and angry but couldn't figure out why she was angry. She answered the oncologist in monosyllables and signed the consent for the chemotherapy quickly. She wanted to start immediately and was pleased when she learned that she'd have her first treatment in two days. The nurse gave her an information package and went through the contents with her. She explained that while Jen was having chemotherapy, she should make sure that she and her husband used condoms so that he wouldn't be exposed to the chemotherapy through her vaginal secretions. Jen reacted to this by closing her eyes and shaking her head. The nurse misinterpreted this and said in a soft voice, "I know this is hard to take. I know just how you're feeling." This was more than Jen could bear. She jumped out of her chair and stormed out of the room. How could anyone know how she was feeling? Her anger erupted, and she barely found her car in the parking garage. She drove home paying no attention to the speed limit, muttering under her breath, and yelling at cars that got in her way.

Noreen was watering the plants in the front of the house when Jen peeled into the driveway. She braked harshly, and a spray of gravel scattered over the grass. Noreen stood there, her mouth open in amazement. What had happened? She didn't have to wait long to hear all about it. The forms, the condescending nurse, and the condoms—it was as if a door had opened and all this stuff was spilling out. Noreen listened. She didn't say anything. She just listened.

Take-Away Points

- Don't ask, don't tell is a dangerous policy, especially in health care.
- Healthcare providers should ask open-ended questions that are inclusive so that gays and lesbians do not feel excluded.
- Using words such as "partner" or "him or her" allows the gay or lesbian patient to walk through the open door and disclose their status.

Dr. Katz Explains

Jen reacted to the global heterosexism found in our society. *Heterosexism* refers to the pervasive attitude in our society that everyone is heterosexual. Forms offer limited options if you are in a same-sex relationship: the choices are single, married, widowed, or divorced. How does someone like Jen fit into these options? She also reacted to the assumption on the part of the nurse that Jen had a husband who would need to use condoms. Now, Jen is in part to blame, as she had not told the nurse that she was in a same-sex relationship. Hopefully, if she had, the nurse would have adapted the information and told her about using a latex barrier for oral sex. But instead, Jen grew angry and left the appointment. It didn't help that the nurse claimed to know what Jen was feeling; she couldn't have been any further from the truth.

Noreen Takes Charge

As Noreen listened to Jen describe her experience, she grew angry, too. But anger was not going to be helpful at this time. When Jen eventually grew quiet, Noreen took her by the hand, and they sat down on a bench under the great oak tree in their front yard. She told Jen just to listen, and this is what she said: "You've done this alone up until now. And I've let you. You cut me out, and I stood by helpless. But from now on, things are going to be different. I'm going to be there with you. Every day. Every appointment. The staff is going to know that you're not alone and that there's someone who loves you, lives with you, and who's got your back. Every day. I do know how you feel. And you were there when I went through this, and I want to be there for you." Jen's whole body reacted to this declaration. She surrendered, and, in that, found strength.

Dr. Katz Explains

At last Noreen stood up and took charge. Sometimes this has to happen and can be difficult when you're trying to respect your partner and how she is managing things. But Jen was obviously not doing well doing things her own way. And Noreen stepped into the fray and took charge this time. Just in time.

We Are Family

When Jen started chemotherapy two days later, Noreen was with her. The nursing staff showed no reaction when the two of them checked in and went together into the treatment area. The nurse who started the IV did ask to be introduced to Jen's "friend," and Noreen interjected, "I'm her partner, and I'm going to be here for all her appointments." The nurse smiled and said that she was pleased to meet her, adding how important it was to have family with you when you're going through treatment. And it is.

CHAPTER 11

Fertility Problems

We were talking about starting a family when this happened.

Fertility issues are important to younger adults when they have to undergo cancer treatment. They're often forced to make difficult decisions at a time when the threat to life is foremost in their minds. And, in the aftermath of treatment, uncertainty exists about getting pregnant. Many people assume that infertility treatment is highly effective and that pregnancy is possible after cancer treatment. The reality is not that simple.

This chapter tells the story of Ruth, who was 24 years old and had just moved in with her boyfriend, Brad, when she was diagnosed with leukemia. They had been dating for four years when this happened and had planned on having a large family. In the chaotic period of diagnosis and beginning treatment, this young couple had to face important issues about fertility. And the aftermath of infertility left more than one victim.

In this chapter, you will learn

- How chemotherapy can affect fertility
- How fertility treatments affect relationships
- How some couples struggle with infertility.

Ruth's Story

Ruth and Brad have been dating for four years. They met at college and discovered that they'd grown up just five miles apart in rural Nebraska. After college, they moved to Omaha, where Brad works as an IT analyst for a bank, and Ruth is an elementary school teacher. They plan to get married next summer, and this past spring they moved in together.

This was a big move for both of them; they come from conservative families, but it just seemed so silly for each of them to be paying rent on separate apartments. Their parents weren't happy but accepted it; they're getting married next year, after all. Ruth is so excited about their little apartment. She spent the summer painting and decorating so that it would be perfect. It even has a spare room that she hopes will be for their first baby. She and Brad want to have a large family. She has a twin sister and two younger brothers, and he's the middle child of five. They have visions of a large house on the outskirts of the city where their children, five or maybe six, could romp in the yard with two big Labrador puppies.

Her World Turned on Its Head

About a month before school started, she went to see her family physician for a routine checkup. She'd been feeling tired but chalked it up to the last-minute rushing to get the apartment decorated before the start of school. She also had some bruises on her legs and arms but thought those were from bumping into furniture while painting and moving things. The doctor asked her about the bruises but didn't seem overly concerned. He sent her for some blood tests, but she always has those as part of her checkups.

The next day, there was a call from his office. Dr. Fletcher got right to the point: "There was an abnormality on your blood test, Ruth. Your white cell count was very high, and I think you may have leukemia. You're going to need to see someone at the hospital immediately. This is serious. You need to go there right away. They're waiting for you to get there. I'm really sorry, Ruth." Just like that, her world turned on its head. Suddenly their perfect apartment felt claustrophobic. She called Brad at work and could only say, "Get home right now. I need you."

Dr. Katz Explains

Bruising and fatigue may be a sign of an abnormality in the blood. But a blood test that shows abnormally high numbers of white blood cells is cause for alarm. Ruth will need further tests, but there is no time to waste; acute leukemia can be life-threatening, and she needs medical attention immediately. As we have seen with the other stories in this book, hearing that you may have cancer comes as a great shock, and most people don't know what questions to ask of their healthcare providers.

The Shock of Discovery

Ruth and Brad sped across town to the hospital. Neither of them said much; Ruth was trying not to cry, and Brad just focused on getting them there in one piece. His head was full of questions, and his heart was beating hard in his chest. This crisis had come out of nowhere, and truth be told, he was terrified. They parked the car and rushed up to the Information Desk. Brad talked for Ruth; he could see she was on the edge of tears and needed to do something, anything, to make her feel better. The woman at the Information Desk directed them down the hall to the Admitting Desk, and there a kindly older woman took over. She asked just a few questions, typed something into the computer, and told them to go to the sixth floor, where Ruth would be admitted immediately. Within 10 minutes, the young couple found themselves in a room with a nurse telling Ruth to put on a hospital gown. Shortly after she did this, a young man in a white coat appeared at the door. He introduced himself as Dr. Cohen and told them he was an oncologist who specialized in hematologic cancers, such as leukemia. At this, Ruth started to sob, and Brad felt tears come to his own eyes. He shook his head and took a deep breath; he needed to be strong to get Ruth through whatever lay ahead.

Dr. Cohen explained that they needed to do a bone marrow biopsy immediately to confirm the diagnosis. Based on the blood test results that he had seen, it was likely acute myeloid leukemia. Ruth was going to need chemotherapy right away and then a stem cell transplant later on. None of this made sense to either of them, but they nodded, and Ruth signed a consent form that was placed in front of her. Minutes later, a nurse came into the room and took Ruth to have the biopsy.

She returned to the room, now her room, about an hour later. They'd taken bone marrow from her hip, and she was quite sleepy from the sedation they'd given her. Later that evening, Dr. Cohen came back to tell them that, as he'd suspected, it was acute myeloid leukemia. Chemotherapy would start in the morning, and she'd be in the hospital for about six weeks. He quietly warned her that the chemotherapy would be hard on her body. He then asked whether they had talked about having children in the future. "Of course we plan to," answered Brad. "We want to have a whole lot of them." Dr. Cohen sat down on the edge of the bed and talked quietly. He explained that the chemotherapy may make it difficult for Ruth to have children. This was more than either of them could bear, and they both started to cry. After a minute or so Ruth asked in a shaky voice, "But isn't there something I could do, like donate my eggs so we could use them later?" Dr. Cohen slowly shook his head. "It's more complicated than that."

Take-Away Points

- The impact of chemotherapy on fertility should be discussed with you, but if it's not, you may have to raise the topic.
- It's important to ask about the impact of any treatment on fertility. Even though the news may not be good, it's better to know so you can make alternate plans if at all possible.
- If treatment doesn't have to start immediately and can wait four to six weeks, it may be possible to have eggs removed from the woman, the eggs fertilized with the partner's sperm, and the embryos frozen.
- Fertility may be affected by chemotherapy depending on the type of drug. Don't assume anything; ask for details.

Dr. Katz Explains

A bone marrow biopsy helps to diagnose leukemia. With the cells that are removed from the bone marrow, the pathologist can provide an accurate picture of what exactly is happening in the body's production of white cells, and from this the correct treatment can be ordered.

Dr. Cohen has asked an important question of this young couple; fertility can be affected by the chemotherapy that is given to destroy the abnormal white cells. Ruth had assumed that she could have eggs removed from her ovaries to then be used sometime in the future to start a pregnancy. But as Dr. Cohen told them, it's not that simple.

Unlike in men, where sperm can be taken and frozen for extended periods of time and then thawed and used to fertilize an egg, it's not that simple for women whose ovaries may be damaged or destroyed by chemotherapy. Eggs just don't freeze all that well, and when they are thawed they generally do not survive. There is a great deal of research going on to solve this problem, including freezing portions of the ovaries that contain eggs or transplanting portions of the ovaries to another part of the body. But this is still experimental, not very successful, and not available in all cities.

One way of getting around this problem is to fertilize some eggs in the laboratory with sperm from the male partner or another donor, allow them to divide, and then freeze the embryos. These can then be implanted into the uterus of the woman or even a surrogate. To do this procedure, the woman would need to take medication that forces a large number of eggs to mature at one time. These eggs would then be removed from her ovaries and mixed with sperm, and the embryos would then be frozen. But this takes time, and Ruth doesn't have time; she needs to start chemotherapy right away.

Time Moves On

Ruth got through the treatment. She stayed in the hospital for the entire six weeks, which passed in a daze. She had all the side effects she was warned about and tried to sleep away the time. Brad visited her every night, and he tried to be supportive but was not really sure what to do to help. Ruth's mother was coming to take care of her when she got out; she would stay in the spare room, which was to be the baby's room.

Two months after she got home, she had the stem cell transplant. Her brother was the donor; he was a good match and was eager to help. Her twin sister really wanted to do it, but their match was too close and the doctors explained that her brother would be better. This time she wasn't the one with the sore hip from the bone marrow extraction. She went back to the hospital for five days of intensive chemotherapy, and then they infused her brother's stem cells into her body.

The most difficult part of this was the isolation; she had to be kept in strict seclusion because her immunity was destroyed by this chemotherapy so that her body would accept the stem cells and start forming healthy cells. She couldn't touch Brad or anyone else for that matter, and anyone who came into her room had to wear a mask, gloves, gown, and head covering. All she could see was their eyes. But it was over, and now she had to wait and see if the stem cells were doing their job.

And Now She's Okay

Eighteen months later, Ruth was almost back to normal. She remembered that period of her life with pain. There was a lot of pain, physical and emotional, for her and for Brad, too, but things were getting better. The only positive thing that happened was that they'd gotten married. It was not the wedding she imagined for so long; it was a small and quiet wedding at her parents' home in the country. But it also was a sign of hope because after the difficult times during her treatment, she wasn't sure that she'd even make it. But she did, and they were officially married. She'd gone back to work at the school and even though she felt a bit rusty after almost two years away, the kids were still the same—noisy and curious—and her days were filled with their needs and demands.

Never far from her thoughts was the desire to have her own children one day. But she remembered Dr. Cohen's face when he told her about the chemotherapy, and for her that was a closed book. Dr. Cohen had told them that her fertility may be affected by the chemotherapy, but there could still be hope. She and Brad haven't talked about that a lot; he hasn't raised the topic, and neither has she. But she thought about it a lot. And so at her next appointment at the hospital, she asked the nurse, who talked to the doctor, who then referred her to a fertility specialist.

Dr. Katz Explains

In the crisis surrounding the diagnosis of a life-threatening illness, many people don't hear the details of what they're told. Ruth heard Dr. Cohen say that her fertility would be affected, so she assumed the worst. But perhaps there was hope, and by asking about it, she was referred to a fertility specialist, who is the right person to work with for this problem.

Ruth's desire for children also is a sign that she is moving to the next phase of the cancer journey—that of survivorship—where the person's hopes and dreams for a normal life take over from the fears and doubts of the period of active treatment.

> ### Take-Away Points
>
> - Ask your healthcare providers for a special appointment after treatment is over to review the exact types of treatment(s) you had and their side effects. You may not have heard or understood everything you were told at the time of diagnosis and treatment.
> - There are no stupid questions, and you have a right to ask about anything and everything, and your healthcare providers have a responsibility to ensure that you have all the information you need to make decisions and to understand what has happened.
> - Ask for a referral to a specialist if you have questions about fertility at any point in the diagnosis and treatment process; they are experts in fertility and can work with the oncology team to maximize your chances of conceiving after treatment.

Hope Rising

Ruth and Brad went to the appointment with the fertility specialist with hope in their hearts but also a great deal of caution. They'd talked of little else since she was referred to this specialist, and while this is the first sign of hope for her and she was really excited, Brad was more controlled and wanted her to be careful and not get her hopes up. The offices where the fertility specialist saw patients were lovely and quite different from the hospital where Ruth had her treatment. The magazines in the waiting room were new, and there was a large fish tank with colorful fish swimming around. She didn't even have to wait very long and was soon called into an office.

A middle-aged man stood up and introduced himself as Dr. Joseph. Without much preamble, he told the couple that he had reviewed the notes from her oncologist and had a few questions for Ruth and Brad. He first asked if her menstrual cycle had returned, and Ruth answered that she'd had her period twice, but there was a six-week gap between the two periods. Dr. Joseph nodded and wrote something in her chart. He asked some more questions about her menstrual cycle before the cancer and then told Ruth that she needed to have some blood tests that would give him information about her hormonal levels. He asked her to make another appointment for early next week and sent her down the hall to a medical lab where three tubes of blood were drawn. As they left the office, Ruth turned to him with a plea in her eyes and her heart: "We were talking about starting a family when this happened. Please help us!"

Ruth left the building with tears in her eyes; for the first time she felt real hope. Brad was also feeling hopeful and allowed himself to imagine the life they wanted to have.

Dr. Katz Explains

The fact that Ruth's periods had come back was a good sign. But they were not regular, which could indicate that she was not ovulating regularly. The results of the blood tests would give the fertility specialist more information.

Most oncologists prefer patients with cancer to wait two to five years after treatment before trying to conceive. This is, in part, because most recurrence occurs within that time frame. If Ruth were pregnant and had a recurrence, she might lose the pregnancy or have to delay treatment, which could jeopardize her chances of success with treatment.

If at First You Don't Succeed . . .

The next week, Ruth and Brad returned to the fertility specialist's office. He had good news for them; the blood tests suggested that Ruth should be able to get pregnant. Ruth was overjoyed and started to cry. These were the first tears of joy she has shed in so many years. He told them to go home and try to make a baby. Brad blushed when he heard this; despite his age he's quite shy about all this and didn't find it easy to talk about sex, even to Ruth.

And so the young couple went home and tried to make a baby. And they tried and then tried some more. Because her periods had not been regular, Ruth was never sure when her period was late, and she spent a lot of money on home pregnancy tests with many false hopes and real disappointments. After six months of this they were getting frustrated. Ruth had been reading about maximizing fertility on a number of Web sites and had all sorts of instructions for Brad. He had to wear boxers and not briefs. He had to follow a certain diet to increase his sperm count. They had to have sex every 48 hours. She had to lie on a pillow with her hips raised after sex. The list went on and on, and Brad didn't like any of it. Sex was regimented, and Ruth was bossy about it. This felt like work and not love, and after six months he wasn't sure how much more he could take.

Dr. Katz Explains

There's a lot of information (and misinformation) about fertility and getting pregnant. There's no evidence to support lying with your hips raised after sex. It does make a difference if the man wears boxers, which allow the testicles to stay away from the body; this may protect the sperm from the heat of the body. And diets don't help, but quitting smoking and not drinking alcohol can help.

Many couples get really stressed about conceiving, and sex becomes a chore and no fun at all. This is natural but not good. Sex really should be loving and fun and pleasurable, and all the rules and instructions take that away.

Take-Away Points

- Be careful about where you get your information. Just because it's published on the Web doesn't mean the information is good or accurate.
- Ask your doctor or fertility specialist for advice.
- Remember that after cancer, you aren't the same as a woman who has not had cancer treatment. It may be much harder for a woman who's had cancer to get pregnant.
- Try to relax even though this is stressful. Stress really makes things worse and may even prevent conception.

When Nothing Seems to Work

Brad and Ruth went back to the fertility specialist. He listened to Ruth's tale of frustration and lost hope. He was sympathetic and told them that if they wanted, they could get more aggressive with the treatment. But this was going to cost a lot of money, and he wanted them to go home and read the package of information that he would give them. Ruth wanted to do something right then; in fact, she was willing to do something at that very appointment. But Brad put his hand over hers and asked her to just go home with him, read the information, and think about it. Ruth did not appreciate this and left the office in a huff. She didn't talk to Brad on the way home and got out of the car quickly and went into the bathroom, where she remained for 45 minutes. Brad just waited it out.

When she came out of the bathroom, her face was streaked with tears and her eyes were red and swollen. "I want this so much," she whispered to him. "You wanted it too. What changed?" Brad quietly explained to her that nothing had changed and he still wanted children, lots of them, if they were blessed to have more than one. But he was worried about her health and didn't want her to have to suffer ever again after all that she had been through with the cancer. Ruth thought about this for a moment and then told him that having children, whatever it took, would never cause her suffering. That's how she saw it, and she was willing to do whatever it took. Brad gave in.

Take-Away Points	Dr. Katz Explains
• Take your time deciding about what you want to do and how far you want to go with assisted reproductive technology. • Consider the costs, both financial and to your health, that accompany these new methods of getting pregnant. • Keep talking to each other about your feelings; some couples break up in the aftermath of failure to conceive.	Many couples set different priorities about having children or the urgency with which they want that to happen. Ruth and Brad's conflict about this is not unusual. Neither is his concern about her health. There are risks to assisted reproduction, and information about this has been offered to the couple. They do need to read and think about the pros and cons of what can be done. And then there is the cost; these technologies can be very expensive and usually are not covered by health insurance.

How Many Eggs in a Dozen?

Ruth agreed to read the information and was a little surprised to learn about the side effects of some of the treatments to stimulate egg production. She hadn't realized that it might be so uncomfortable. And the cost. But she knew in her heart that it would be worth it. And they could always borrow money from her parents, and her twin sister had offered to help in any way she could.

They went back to Dr. Joseph the next week. They had agreed to try three cycles of treatment, and if that didn't work, they were going to take a break. Brad was not sure that Ruth would keep up her side of the bargain, but what could he do? She really wanted this, and he did too, just not in the same way.

Dr. Joseph explained that Ruth would take drugs to stimulate her ovaries to produce more eggs. This was the first treatment they would try. He instructed them to have intercourse as they normally would; he missed the look that passed between them. Brad was not sure what "normal" intercourse meant anymore.

He could tell that Ruth was really excited to go home and get started, and that's what they did. Ruth had the prescription for the medication in her hand, and they filled it at the drugstore on their way home.

Over the next month, Ruth grew irritable and bloated. She didn't complain, and Brad tried not to, but she was snippy with him, and making love was just not fun. He felt like a performing seal but made sure to hide this from Ruth. He'd complained once when she told him it was time for sex; he'd been raking leaves all afternoon and was tired, but her response was testy to say the least! So he did his duty.

Four days later, he found her crying in the bathroom. She was bleeding. It hadn't worked. He tried to comfort her, but she just kept crying.

Dr. Katz Explains

The drugs that cause multiple eggs to ripen in the ovaries also make women feel bloated and irritable, like a bad case of PMS. Add to this the stress of trying to get pregnant, the cost of the drugs, and having to have sex on certain days, and you have a combination that often causes a great deal of unhappiness. And success is not guaranteed. About 50% of women will get pregnant in the first three cycles on these medications, but that means that 50% will not. And these statistics don't refer to women who've had chemotherapy.

Where Do We Go From Here?

Another month went by, and once again Ruth's period made an appearance. She was getting desperate and had started talking about what to do next. Brad was too scared to remind Ruth that they'd agreed that after three unsuccessful cycles they would take a break. She was determined to get pregnant, and as the days went by, her determination grew. She told Brad she was thinking about quitting her job because perhaps working was stressing her out and preventing her from getting pregnant. Brad couldn't believe his ears! How were they ever going to be able to afford any kind of treatment without her paycheck?

Brad could barely look at the calendar that Ruth had pinned to the bathroom wall. On it in red marker was the days that she had taken the pills and a large question mark over a Saturday when her next period was due. This was only three days away. He caught Ruth feeling her breasts when she thought he wasn't looking. Were they more or less tender? Had they grown bigger? Could this mean something?

And that Saturday he woke to hear her crying in the bathroom once again. He couldn't help feeling a little bit of relief; they'd agreed to a break, and he was looking forward to a couple of months without the pressure of trying to get Ruth pregnant. But this third period just made her resolve even stronger, and the next week he found himself once again in Dr. Joseph's office.

He sat quietly while Ruth and Dr. Joseph discussed the next steps. Suddenly it just burst out of him: "Stop! Ruth, we said we'd wait. We agreed to take a break if it didn't work. Now you're talking about artificial insemination. That wasn't part of the deal."

Take-Away Points
• Emotions are high, and with a 50% chance of failure, disappointment is an expectation.
• Be prepared for feelings of failure and blame, both your own and your partner's.
• It may be helpful to seek some form of counseling both before and during treatment for infertility.

Dr. Katz Explains

Despite agreeing to a plan, this couple now is at odds about what comes next. This is not uncommon, and it is often the woman who lets down her side of the deal. She's the one who has to take the medication and has to suffer the side effects. She's the one who perhaps feels pregnant as the result of the drugs and has to face the disappointment of her body's failure to get pregnant. None of this is logical; it's highly emotional and not rational. But many men look at these things in a much more rational way and don't have the same physical feelings, so it's just not the same for them.

A Bitter Ending

Ruth refused to consider taking a break; it was as if she were on a mission, and nothing and no one was going to stop her. And that included Brad. It was as if she was possessed, and he didn't really recognize the woman she'd become.

Dr. Joseph seemed uncomfortable with the way things were going in his office. Ruth was getting angrier and angrier with Brad, and he was not talking to her. Suddenly Brad got up from his chair and left the room. Ruth looked surprised at this and followed him. She apologized to Dr. Joseph as she ran out the room, and he just shook his head wearily; he'd seen similar couples before.

Ruth tried talking to Brad on the way home, but this time he was not willing to talk. Once again, the ride home was silent. And Brad entered the house and went straight to their room. She left him alone for a few minutes and went to the computer to look up some information about artificial insemination. She heard him coming down the stairs, turned around, and was shocked to see he had a bag in his hands. "Where are you going?" she asked, her voice shaking slightly. "I have to take a break from this, from you," he replied. They both stared at each other for a long moment. She opened her mouth to speak, to plead, to demand that he stay. But she had no words.

CHAPTER 12

Sexuality and Terminal Illness

One last time . . .

It may seem strange to think that women in the terminal stages of cancer have sexual needs and desires. Sex and death just don't seem to go together, and some would say that these are the last remaining taboos in society. We've come a long way in how we think and talk about and care for people in the terminal stages of illness. And we have to come to terms with the fact that even as death nears, there is a need for intimacy and touch that reflects on what has been for the couple.

In this chapter, you will hear Caryl's story. Caryl had terminal ovarian cancer and wanted to stay at home in the final stages of her disease. Her three daughters, now in their teens, wanted to care for their mom, and Caryl didn't want to leave them. Caryl's husband was devastated by what was happening to his wife and drew on their large circle of friends to support and help in the last few weeks of her life.

In this chapter, you will learn that
- Even in the end stages of cancer, women have needs for intimacy.
- Intimacy is possible, even in the midst of end-of-life care.

Caryl's Story

Caryl always had been a fitness enthusiast; she ran track and field in high school and went to college on an athletic scholarship. That's how she met Jeff, her husband of 20 years and the love of her life; he was the quarterback on the football team and also on a scholarship. Their story read like a Harlequin romance; graduation followed by a summer wedding followed by three lovely girls, all of them two years apart. Jeff worked for his dad's car dealership and took over the family business when his dad retired. He was very successful in this, and soon their car dealership was the biggest in the state. They led a comfortable life, and Caryl never worked outside the home. She was active at the girls' schools and involved in book clubs and charity work in their community. She remained athletic and had run three marathons in her 30s but switched to the half-marathon when she turned 40; the long training runs were just too much for her, and she could run the half-marathon with much less training.

Two years ago after one such half-marathon, she felt tired well past the point of when she should have recovered from the race. She also noticed that her pants were feeling tighter, and she had this vague feeling of pressure in her pelvis. She was worried for a while but soon got busy with organizing the library's annual fundraising ball. Then it was Christmas, and they took the girls on a Caribbean cruise. When they returned from the cruise, she noticed that she felt bloated and nauseated a lot of the time, but she put that down to too much rich food on the boat and went on with her life. Four months later, she went for her annual checkup, and her doctor felt something abnormal during her pelvic exam; weeks of testing followed, and she was shocked to learn that she had advanced ovarian cancer. The next few months were a blur of tests and more tests and then surgery followed by chemotherapy.

Dr. Katz Explains

Ovarian cancer frequently has insidious onset with vague sensations like bloating and nausea that are often attributed to something else. This kind of cancer is often diagnosed when it is quite advanced. Surgery and chemotherapy are the most common treatments, but recently, administering chemotherapy directly into the abdominal cavity has been shown to be effective for some women. It's a difficult treatment to get through, and most women feel really sick, and some may not be able to complete all six treatment cycles.

The Depths of Misery

Caryl was one of those women who had severe side effects, and she wasn't able to complete more than three cycles of treatment. She blamed herself for this and apologized to Jeff for being such a failure. He was barely coping with what was happening to her and their family. The girls were withdrawn and at times angry and, for the first time in their lives, were staying out late at night. Jeff suspected that Jen, the middle daughter, was smoking. But he didn't have the energy to deal with it and really didn't know what to do; Caryl had always been the disciplinarian, and he couldn't burden her with this.

Caryl was angry, too. She was angry that this had happened to her after all her efforts at keeping fit and healthy. She was angry that this had happened at a time when her daughters were in their teen years (they ranged in age from 14 to 18) and needed her more than ever. And she was angry that there didn't seem to be much that the doctors could do for her. They'd told her that she wasn't tolerating the chemotherapy in her abdomen and there wasn't much point in trying anything else. All she read about in magazines and saw on TV were the miracle stories—the women who had breast cancer and who then ran marathons and wrote books—and she wasn't going to have a miracle in her life.

In the Dark of Night

Visits to the oncologist were difficult for Caryl. It usually started a few days before the visit when she went for blood tests; these were important because if her C125 levels were down, this was a good sign. But they only went down once in the months since she stopped chemotherapy, and since then, they had risen slowly. Every time she had her blood drawn, her anxiety rose. She couldn't sleep and spent the long nights in front of the TV in the den, not watching but afraid to be in the dark. In those hours, all her worst fears came to the surface; her girls struggling without her, her husband lonely and not coping, and her friends going on without her. These were not rational thoughts, she knew that, but in the dark of the night, they loomed like specters from a bad horror movie. Morning came, and she was exhausted. She seemed to grow thinner by the day, and her normally trim and muscular body was now gaunt. She hid this by wearing sweatsuits and never undressing in front of Jeff. She thought her family members didn't notice, but of course they did.

Dr. Katz Explains

Because ovarian cancer often is diagnosed late, the prognosis may not be good. Many women with this kind of cancer find themselves very angry that this has happened to them. And anticipating the loss for your family also is not unusual or bad. But Caryl seems to be very alone in her struggles even though her family recognizes that things are not going well. Everyone protects one another, so nothing is said. Jeff is struggling to cope, as are their daughters.

The Difficult Conversation

Caryl usually went to her oncology appointments with a friend. She didn't want to bother Jeff and knew it was difficult for him to sit with her in the waiting room. And there was never any good news at the appointments, or so it seemed. So she told him to go to work, and she had a roster of good friends who were more than willing to drive her and wait until she was done. But three days before her next appointment, the nurse from the clinic called and asked her to bring Jeff with her. She heard this request with a sick feeling in her stomach; this could only mean something bad.

At this appointment, it was not just the oncologist who was there; a social worker whom she had not met before also was in the room. The oncologist explained that they'd done everything possible, and there was nothing more to do. Caryl was dying (the first thought that went through her head was "duh!"), and it was time to talk about

Take-Away Points

- Include children in these kinds of important discussions, especially if they are teenagers or older. Children know more than you think they do and often become more confused or anxious if information is withheld from them.
- There are many different options for end-of-life care, including palliative care in a hospice or hospital. But many people want to die at home, and that may be an option.
- Your healthcare team should have information for you about end-of-life care in your area.

end-of-life care. They sat there in shock, and Jeff was particularly devastated. He'd really not thought that this could or would happen; he always found solutions for problems, so why couldn't the oncologist? The social worker talked about palliative care and hospice care, and even though she was obviously good at her job, the words just swirled around the room and didn't reach the couple. They walked slowly back to the car, suddenly older than their years.

That weekend, they read the pamphlets the social worker had provided. And they brought the girls into the conversation. It was time for them to face the truth, and they needed to have a voice, too. Jeff was surprised by their reaction; they seemed to change in an instant from teenagers to young women. "Can you stay at home, mom, please? Can we take care of you?" Caryl started to cry; this is what she wanted but hadn't known how to ask. She wanted to be at home with Jeff and her girls until the end.

Almost at the Finish Line

Caryl's friends proved to be a formidable force; within just a few days of hearing that she had entered the end stages of her cancer, they formed a team that was available to help her and her family in whatever ways they could. It was summer, so her three daughters were home all day. They spent most of their time sitting quietly with Caryl, gauging her energy level and responding to her needs. The friends, lovingly described by Caryl as "her favorite few," kept the fridge and pantry stocked with food and drinks for the many visitors who came around to see Caryl. They also took turns doing the housekeeping, something that amused Caryl very much, as many of them had housekeepers and had never cleaned their own homes. Just the sight of them with a mop or duster was enough to make Caryl giggle, even though that made her breathless. Jeff spent as much time as he could at home, but truthfully, he felt a little outnumbered by the women gathered around Caryl.

Once a week, a nurse from the hospice program at the hospital came to visit. She made sure that Caryl was pain free and offered advice and support to the three daughters, who were doing such a good job caring for their mom. Every day they helped her shower, dried her hair, and put some blush and lip gloss on her. They filed her nails and massaged her feet. Caryl was surrounded by much love and support; the nurse talked to her colleagues about how

Take-Away Points

- Family and friends want to help but often don't know what to do; giving them tasks (cleaning, doing laundry or dishes) can be both helpful and make them feel useful.
- Moving to a central part of the house can be convenient, but it also can be tiring as you are in the middle of all the action and may have little down time.
- Friends sometimes take over, and this may exclude spouses and family members; as a friend, take your lead from family members and ask if you're overstepping your bounds.

sometimes, even under the worst circumstances, things can be pretty near perfect.

As the weeks passed, the nurse noticed that Caryl seemed more exhausted and was experiencing more pain. She sat down next to Caryl's bed and talked to her about moving a bed into the den so she wouldn't have to climb the stairs, something that was becoming too much for her in her weakened state. She also offered her more medication to control the pain and the anxiety that Caryl felt during the night when she couldn't sleep. These all seemed like good ideas, and within a couple of hours, a hospital bed had arrived at the house and was installed in the den. Caryl's friends made a point of bringing flowers from their gardens, and the room glowed with their color and beauty.

Personal Privacy

Caryl passed most days in a dreamlike state. She was neither hungry nor thirsty, and her anger had disappeared. It had been replaced by a sense of peace and a strange sort of happiness in watching her daughters spend time with her. But Jeff seemed to be missing, and she was not sure how to find him. He came in and out of the den but seemed like a deer caught in the headlights. All her needs were obviously being taken care of, and he was not sure what to do or how he could contribute. One afternoon the nurse from the hospice noticed that he was on the edge of the activity around Caryl, and she took him aside. "You seem sort of left out," she suggested quietly, and Jeff nodded his head. Tears welled in his eyes and he seemed hesitant to speak. "Why don't I let you guys have some privacy?" asked the nurse, and he just nodded again, more vigorously this time.

She went into the room and quietly asked the girls and the two friends who were there to give Caryl and Jeff some time alone. The girls looked embarrassed and quickly left the room. Caryl's friends left as well, their concern spread over their faces—was this the end?—but they realized that the couple needed some time alone. As they left the room, Jeff drew the nurse aside. "Can I touch her?" he asked hesitantly. "I miss her so much, and she's still here." His voice cracked and he shook his head, willing the feelings away. The nurse answered, "Of course you can touch her. I bet she'd love that and misses it, too." The nurse left the house, stopping in the kitchen to remind the girls that they were doing an excellent job in caring for their mom.

Dr. Katz Explains

Even though having the dying person in the middle of the house, in this case the den, makes caring for her easier and more comfortable, it also means that privacy is lost. Being in the middle of the comings and goings also can be exhausting.

Jeff asked the nurse if he could touch his wife; this may not mean sexual touching, but often in the changed reality of this end-of-life stage, spouses may feel that they need permission to touch their loved ones or may be worried that they may hurt them. And it may be that he does want to touch her in a more sexual way; this does not mean that he wants to have intercourse with her but that he wants to feel her body next to his, perhaps for the last time. For many couples, sex is a way of expressing love and affection and gratitude, and at the end of life, the need to express those emotions does not disappear. The couple just needs to find a comfortable way of doing that.

A Final Encounter

The house was strangely quiet when the nurse and Caryl's friends left. The girls had gone up to their rooms, and Jeff could hear the sound of music through their bedroom doors. He approached the hospital bed slowly, and Caryl opened her eyes at the sound of his footsteps. She smiled at the sight of him, this man that she had loved since she was 19, and she beckoned to him to come closer. "Wanna fool around?" she whispered, their code phrase of invitation to each other. Jeff's response scared them both; he started to sob as men do, loudly and messily. She slowly shifted her emaciated body in the bed, making room for her husband of 20 years. He lay down next to her carefully, his tears falling onto her shoulder. She brushed the hair off his face and looked into his eyes. "I meant it.

Wanna fool around?" Jeff was not sure what she meant. How could she possibly be thinking about sex? Was she joking? Was he hearing things? She repeated herself, more insistent this time. "Wanna fool around? One last time?" Her hand pulled at his sleeve and she seemed to want him to get on top of her. Jeff held his breath and did what she told him to. Resting carefully on his elbows and knees, he held himself over her. He dared not put any of his weight on her; she was so thin she barely made a bump under the sheets. She poked him in the ribs, "You just going to stay there all night?" So softly, so softly it felt like a whisper, he moved across and up and down her body. His body hovered over hers, not touching, in a poignant imitation of what they had done so many times before. The sheets barely stirred under him, his weight on her was so light, and after just a minute he moved back down next to her. A deep sigh ruffled his hair, and he could feel her smile as she said the words she'd said so many times, "That was the best sex I ever had." And she fell asleep in his arms, perhaps for the last time.

Dr. Katz Explains

Expressing love takes many forms, and in this encounter, there is true intimacy, as soft as a whisper and as close as a breath. In this encounter, Caryl led the way and told her husband what to do. This was a gift for them both, so different from what had gone on before but so special in its remembrances of times past.

She Left in the Morning

Two days later, the nurse told Jeff that the end could come at any time. Caryl was barely conscious anymore and yet her spirit filled the house. Her friends still came by every day, but they mostly stayed in the kitchen, talking quietly and making tea or coffee for themselves. Jeff had started to sleep on the couch in the den, and the girls took turns sitting with Caryl if he dozed.

As the sky lightened in the predawn hours, the girls were all in their beds. Jeff was asleep, and something in the air made him open his eyes. He didn't even have to touch her; he knew she had left.

PART THREE

Seeking Help

In this section, you'll learn about useful resources and strategies to get you on the road to sexual recovery. You'll also learn what happens to a partner of a woman with cancer and how he developed sexual problems of his own when his wife had problems after cancer.

CHAPTER 13

Lotions and Potions

What medications or treatments are helpful for cancer survivors who are experiencing sexual difficulties? Can we believe what we read and see on television, on the Internet, and in magazines? All sorts of pharmaceutical and nonpharmaceutical products are available that are suggested to help with lowered libido, decreased arousal, and altered sensations of orgasms. This chapter presents information about what may work and what won't, what's helpful and safe, and what's untested and potentially harmful.

Let's start with products that claim to increase **libido or sexual interest.** As discussed in previous chapters, libido is a complex phenomenon that is partly psychological and partly cognitive. Basically, it's all in your head. And in your heart, too. A lot has been written about the use of testosterone to improve libido in women. As you may recall, testosterone is a sex hormone and often is described as a male hormone. Women have low levels of testosterone that are produced in the ovaries and in the adrenal glands that lie on top of the kidneys. We don't know what levels of this hormone are normal for women, and some studies have suggested that levels of testosterone and sexual interest are not connected in women.

We do know that women who have had their ovaries removed (which happens often when you have a hysterectomy) before they go through menopause and are given testosterone do show some improvements in feelings of general well-being and perhaps also in sexual functioning. In two trials of a testosterone patch in women, the number of satisfying sexual episodes (the measured outcome in the studies) increased from 0.5 and 0.73 episodes in four weeks to 2.1 and

1.56 episodes in four weeks in each of two trials. There was also a strong placebo effect; women in the control group on the placebo patch that contained no drug were as likely to report an increase in the number of sexual episodes. And the trials continued for only six weeks. In real life, women would use these patches for much longer, and the safety of this could not be established from these short trials.

Testosterone also is converted to estrogen in the fatty tissue of our bodies, so women with breast cancer should not take testosterone because this can increase their risk of having a recurrence. It also should be used with caution in women with other kinds of cancer until its safety is proven for use in this population.

Other products are advertised to increase **arousal or sexual excitement**. Many over-the-counter products contain substances that are irritating (such as peppermint oil) that cause increased blood flow to the surface of the skin or mucous membranes. This blood flow could be interpreted as arousal. It also may be that the act of applying the product to the genital area is what increases arousal. Most of these products instruct the user to rub the substance into the area very well, and it may be the rubbing that increases arousal and not the product. Read the labels carefully; if you see borage oil, peppermint oil, or any other "natural" ingredient that may irritate tissues, then stay away from it. If the label warns you to keep the substance out of your eyes, this is a clear warning that it should not touch your genitals either. This is particularly important for women who have had radiation to their genital area, as the tissues will be sensitive.

Vaginal dryness is a common problem for women who either have had their ovaries surgically removed or are on medication that suppresses hormone production. A number of strategies can help with this. Some over-the-counter products may be helpful. The first is a vaginal moisturizer such as Replens® ('Lil Drug Store Products, Inc.). This is a product that increases the amount of natural lubricant in the vaginal walls by trapping up to 60 times its weight in water, which is then captured in the tissues of the vagina. This product is generally used up to three times a week and can keep you feeling more comfortable if you are experiencing pain from vaginal dryness. It is not intended to make vaginal penetration more comfortable during sexual activity, although this does occur for some women. You need to use it for a period of three to four weeks to see best results. After that, you can cut back on use, and with trial and error you'll find how often you need to use it to stay comfortable.

A vaginal moisturizer will not solve the underlying cause of vaginal dryness, which is a result of decreased estrogen levels. To change this, you need to use either a local or a systemic formulation of estrogen, such as an estrogen cream, pill, or ring. When used locally in the form of a cream, an estrogen pessary, or a ring containing estrogen that is placed in the vagina, estrogen is only absorbed into the general circulation in very small amounts. Your oncologist may have an opinion about whether you can be exposed to even the tiniest amount of estrogen, and you need to discuss this with him or her. But this is the most effective treatment for vaginal dryness.

Lubricants are products designed to make vaginal penetration more comfortable. They can be used for sexual activity and also when you have to use a dilator after radiation therapy. A number of these are available at the drugstore or supermarket and most of these are water-based. The most well-known of these is K-Y® Jelly (McNeil-PPC, Inc.), which is used just before sexual activity. Some women find that it dries out quite quickly during intercourse and gets sticky. An alternative is a lubricant called Astroglide® (Biofilm, Inc.). This glycerin-based product does not get sticky even after prolonged use and can be replenished with water. Some women find that the glycerin increases their risk of getting a vaginal yeast infection. Both of these products now are available in a warming variety, which can add some spice to sex play.

Silicone lubricants stay fluid much longer and are not absorbed by the skin. Any residue left behind needs to be cleaned off with soap and water, and the silicone can be slippery on wet bathroom surfaces. These lubricants cause deterioration of silicone dilators or sex toys and therefore should not be used with these. Silicone lubricants generally are not available in drugstores but can be found in sex stores or online (such as at www.blowfish.com).

Oil-based lubricants, such as petroleum jelly, generally are not recommended. They destroy latex condoms. Some women use olive oil, coconut oil, vitamin E oil, or cocoa butter. Clear mineral oil may be used, as well, but it often contains petroleum and therefore should be used with caution.

For women who are having difficulties with **orgasms**, learning new ways of stimulating themselves or teaching their partner may help. A number of books are recommended in Chapter 16 that may provide helpful information. Many women find that using a vibrator gives them orgasms that are reliable and intense. There's no need to even go to a sex store to buy one; you can use any handheld wand massager or vibrator to achieve the same goal. Experiment with the amount of pressure you use, where the vibrator is placed (directly on the clitoris or slightly above, below, or to the side), and whether there is fabric over the clitoris or not. Some women find the sensation too intense when the vibrator is placed directly on the clitoris without some fabric to protect it.

Conclusion

This chapter is not intended to endorse or promote any product or service. As with any product, the principle of "buyer beware" applies. Before using anything on your genital area or taking any medication, prescribed or over-the-counter, natural or organic, be sure to check with your healthcare provider. This is especially important when you're having active treatment.

CHAPTER 14

Talking About Sex

Strategies to Ease the Tension

It's often said that the biggest sex organ is the brain, and if that's true—and why wouldn't it be—then the eyes and mouth are the runners-up. Not in size perhaps, but certainly in importance. They're really close to the brain and have direct and instant communication with it. And they say eyes see things that both stimulate our senses and our sexual organs, while the mouth talks and says things that can both improve and destroy our relationships.

This chapter focuses on communication, which is an important part of our everyday lives and essential to our relationships. Talking about sex is not easy for many of us; we may joke about it, and sex is a source of humor from childhood on, but meaningful talk about sex, especially with our partner, is more difficult and may be a source of pain and frustration for many of us.

Why is it so difficult to talk about sex? Everyone else seems to talk about it. On television, talk show hosts chat about it all the time. The music channels have songs about it, using slang terms and rude gestures. The tabloids report on the sex lives of celebrities and politicians. But is any of this talk meaningful? No, and there's the problem. We don't hear many meaningful discussions about sex, so we don't know how to have those conversations ourselves.

Most of us have been influenced by generations of negative messages about sex: nice girls don't, boys have to have it, and it can get you in trouble. Most of us never had any decent sex education. If we were lucky, we learned about menstruation and hygiene products but nothing about sexual pleasure and negotiation of what we need and want to have that pleasure. Many of us didn't have any healthy sexual role models; our parents didn't talk about sex other than to warn us of what might happen if we were bad girls. And many of us have never learned the words to describe our sexual parts and how to use them to experience pleasure. Many of us have never learned what brings us pleasure and have relied on our partners to give us pleasure even if they also were affected by the same negativity and ignorance. Many of us may still believe that masturbation is a sin. Or that it will make you crazy and grow hair on your palms. And go blind. If that were true, there'd be millions and millions of blind people walking around and there'd be salons where we could go to get the hair on our palms styled and cut.

All of these factors contribute to our difficulty talking about sex. These same factors influence our healthcare providers, and that's one reason why they may not be talking to you about sex and cancer. Or it may reflect the small amount of time devoted to the study of human sexuality in their education programs in nursing and medical school. It's a real pity.

But perhaps the biggest barrier to meaningful conversation about sex is that we are afraid. We're afraid of saying the wrong thing and making fools of ourselves. We're afraid of hurting or insulting our partner. We're afraid of saying something that could anger our partner or make him or her feel threatened. And we're afraid that we may be rejected if we say what we really feel.

Here are some suggestions to help you and your partner talk about sex and love and passion and pain and anything else that is getting in the way of your relationship.

Find the time.

Just like any other important discussion you've ever had, you need to set aside time to talk about sex. This is not a conversation you should have while rushing to get to work. You probably find the time to plan a vacation, right? So find the time to talk about this important part of your relationship. Any problems you may be having did not start overnight, and they're not going to be solved overnight, either. So when you do talk, remember to plan to talk again and soon. But set limits for how long you are going to talk, and when the conversation is over, it's over and should not be strung out over days and weeks.

And when you're planning the time to talk, plan the place as well. Strange as this may sound, talking about sex shouldn't happen in the bedroom (or any other place where you have sex). Find a neutral place and turn off the TV, the stereo, and the phone. Lock the front door. Make sure the dog has food and water and has been out for a walk. Interruptions can make a sensitive topic seem even more overwhelming and may break the flow of the discussion or may distract one or both of you from the task at hand.

Say the words.

Many of us have a "down there" . . . really our vulva and vagina and other parts associated with sex and reproduction. But we've never said those words aloud and perhaps have never even heard them said aloud. And male parts may be even stranger to say! Some of us may only know the cute baby words we heard from our parents when we were young and then used with our own kids. But we feel embarrassed to use them when talking to our partners.

Try saying one of these words out loud: "vagina." Then say it again. And again. It gets easier all the time!

Name the problem.

You need to decide ahead of time what you want to talk about. And you need to be prepared to discuss it openly and honestly and constructively. This requires planning ahead, and it's a good idea to let your partner know what you want to talk about. Saying "Honey, we need to talk about our sex life" is too broad and may be confusing to him or her. What about your sex life? The frequency, the type of activity, your feelings about it? Be clear with your partner so that he or she also can do some thinking ahead of time. A better invitation may be "I would like to talk about the pain I have during intercourse."

Practice straight talk.

Talking about sex requires you to be clear in your words and expectations. Many of us think that our partner can or should be able to guess or intuitively know our needs and feelings. You may know each other very well, and you may be able to finish each others' sentences, and you may even think the same things at the same time, but if you want to solve a problem, then you need to be straightforward and clear about what you are thinking and feeling.

Tell your partner what you are feeling and why this is happening. The context is very important to avoid your partner thinking that the reason you are feeling this way is something that he or she has done. A vague statement, such as "I have no desire for sex," may be interpreted as "She doesn't love/want me anymore," when what you mean is that since your chemotherapy, you're very tired, your vagina hurts, and you'd rather kiss and cuddle.

Use the "I" word.

It's very important to talk about yourself and not put words in the mouth of your partner. That's just not fair, and it won't help your conversation. If you need more direct stimulation since your surgery to get aroused, say something like "I would love it if you would touch my clitoris with a little more pressure. Let me show you how I like it." That's much more constructive than "You don't know how to get me excited."

By talking in "I" statements, you take ownership of your own feelings and don't put words in your partner's mouth or assume that you know what he or she is thinking or feeling. And from your partner's perspective, it doesn't feel like blame.

Balance the negative and the positive.

There are different ways of saying things, and how you say something can strongly influence how the message is received. "You make me crazy with your demands for sex" has a very different tone than "I don't want sex as often as you seem to." Sometimes in talking about sex, we have to say things that may seem hurtful or may appear to our partner as criticism. Balancing the positive and the negative is a delicate task, but if done carefully, it can protect feelings and reduce the risk of causing hurt. If you find that your response to your partner's caress has changed, instead of stating the negative ("You don't know how to make me feel good"), you can be positive by stating "Let me show you where to touch me so that it feels really good."

Listen.

When your partner speaks, make the effort to listen, with both your ears and your heart and mind. Don't think about the laundry, what you have to do tomorrow, or that he's said that same thing before. Empty your mind of past memories and future plans and truly listen.

Some couples find it useful to have a small item, such as a wooden spoon or other knickknack, for the person who's talking to hold. When he's holding the item, it is his turn to talk, and he must not be interrupted until he gives the item to the other person. This can help to focus the listener's attention because he or she cannot talk while the other person has the item.

One of the greatest gifts we can experience in our relationship is to be truly heard. So think about giving that gift to your partner by listening with your heart, mind, and soul.

Be flexible.

You may want something to be resolved in a certain way, but your partner may have different views. When talking about important subjects we sometimes get defensive and stubborn, and then nothing gets resolved. Give a little. When you are actively listening to your partner, let go of your own thoughts and opinions for a moment or two, and you may be surprised that your partner's position is not that far from yours.

Get help.

Don't wait until you're faced with a crisis to get help. If every discussion ends up in a fight, you may need help. If every fight ends up with a week of silence, you need help. Marriage therapists and sex therapists or counselors are highly educated professionals who specialize in helping couples to understand what is affecting their relationship and, more importantly, helping them to find a better way of talking or reacting or loving.

Communication is central to all our relationships. But we all need practice in getting it right.

CHAPTER 15

Male Sexual Difficulties

What happens to one partner when the other gets cancer?

When one member of a couple is affected by cancer, the partner suffers, too. This chapter will detail some specific sexual issues that can have an impact on the partner. For example, some men may experience erectile difficulties in response to the pain or altered sensations with sex that their partners are experiencing.

In this chapter, you'll meet Gayle and Dave, a couple in their mid 60s that were enjoying retirement until Gayle was diagnosed with uterine (endometrial) cancer. Her treatment included surgery and radiation. While her prognosis was good, Gayle has struggled with sexual difficulties that also affected Dave's sexual functioning.

Unlike the other chapters in this book, the focus of this chapter is on the man, and you'll learn

- How men's sexual functioning can be altered by their partner's sexual problems
- Some strategies to address these issues.

Dave's Story

When he stopped to think about it, Dave couldn't believe how difficult the last year had been. His wife, Gayle, was treated for uterine cancer in early January. Just when things were going well for the couple (they'd both recently retired), that had to happen! She was in the hospital for five days when she had the surgery, and it took her a really long time to recover after that. Dave was not used to doing things around the house, and he found it difficult to keep things going during that time. And six weeks after that, just when she was starting to feel better, she had to have the radiation treatments, and that made her very tired. That made him grumpy. He wanted things to be the way they were before; they had such great plans for their retirement—golf and winters in Florida. But that's all gone now. When he thought of the future, he just felt down. This was definitely *not* what he'd planned.

Dr. Katz Explains

Cancer affects more than just the person who has the cancer. It also can have a significant effect on the partner and other family members. Dave finds himself in the position of having his carefully planned retirement changed. And he's not happy. This may seem selfish, and perhaps it is, but some people have less resilience than others, and some people, like Dave, just don't do well when things happen that ruin their plans.

Partners sometimes experience depression and anxiety when their partners get sick. This is not a cry for attention but a very real response to a change and challenge in their lives. But when all the attention is focused on the person with cancer, the partner's needs may go unattended, and this may have serious effects.

The Sun Comes Up Again

Almost exactly one year after Gayle's surgery, Dave could see a change in her. She had more energy and seemed interested in getting out more. She even started to take an interest in cooking again, and Dave was really excited about that. He'd been living on sandwiches and soup for most of the year and could do with her home cooking again.

She even seemed more interested in him. For the past year, she'd avoided him most of the time, especially when he tried to put his arm around her. In the beginning she'd push his arm away and make a "pshaw" kind of noise out of her nose. But after her radiation treatment, she just kept out of arm's reach.

He'd talked to a couple of his friends about this; some of their wives had also had hysterectomies, and they told him in no uncertain terms that sex was a distant memory after that.

But she definitely seemed more interested in him recently. She hadn't made any sexual advances toward him, that was not her style, but she seemed softer with him, and last night after dinner, she'd patted him on the head. That was a good sign. They'd slept in different rooms since her surgery. She found it difficult to sleep, and she said his snoring was enough to deafen half the people in the building. He didn't hear himself snore, so he did not argue with her on this one.

Dr. Katz Explains

Individuals and couples all have established patterns of behavior when it comes to sexuality; these are called *sexual scripts*. These may be quite rigid in that some people or couples are always sexual in the same way. Think about how you are as a sexual being. Is your sex life creative and inventive? Do you like novelty or do you prefer to do the same thing(s) over and over again? There is no right or wrong with sexual scripts; they are what they are.

Dave and Gayle's sexual script is a fairly traditional one. He initiates, and she either agrees or refuses. She's been doing a lot more refusing since she got sick. She sends him messages, like patting him on the head, which has special meaning for them. In this case, it may mean that she's interested, but he must still make the first move.

Maybe Tonight . . .

Dave had followed Gayle onto the deck after she patted him on the head. He was not going to miss his chance. He carefully put his arm around her waist, and she didn't move or push his arm away. Dave couldn't believe his luck. He kissed her on the side of her neck and still she stayed there. Dave could barely breathe and quickly took her hand and led her to the bedroom. He had to think about which bedroom to go to now that they were sleeping separately. Gayle started to chuckle, "The one with the big bed, silly," and they went to the bedroom they had shared for 42 years, excluding the last one.

Dave and Gayle were soon moving in the same way that they had for 43 years, not counting the two years of their courtship. Gayle seemed to be aroused, and Dave was so excited that he didn't spend as much time on foreplay as he used to. Part of his brain was telling him to slow down, but other parts were telling him to go full speed ahead in case she changed her mind. As he tried to insert his penis into her vagina he felt her stiffen and then he heard her take in a quick, sharp breath. He suddenly realized that he might be hurting her and tried to stop and say something . . . but instead he climaxed, and, just like that, it was over.

Dr. Katz Explains

What happened to Dave is not unusual. He was so aroused after all that time that he got carried away. He didn't spend as much time on foreplay as he should have and used to, and he didn't ask her if she was ready for intercourse. When he tried to penetrate her, she reacted (with pain? or surprise?), and this interfered with his reaction, and he had an orgasm, much sooner than he wanted to.

In medical terms this would be called *premature, rapid,* or *early ejaculation.* It is not an illness, and unless it bothers the man or his partner, there is no need to seek treatment. But it may bother one or both of them.

The Aftermath

Dave moved off her and lay down next to her. He was afraid to speak and so he just lay there with his eyes closed, every now and then sneaking a glance at Gayle. She was lying there too, but the second time he glanced at her he saw a tear inching down her cheek. Dave hated to see Gayle cry. It really bothered him. And this time it prompted him to speak: "I'm sorry, love. Did I hurt you? What did I do wrong?" Gayle burst into tears. She told him that she'd felt so bad this past year, denying him sex and seeing him so frustrated. Dave tried to stop her; he wanted to tell her it was all right and that his friends had told him that it was normal to not have sex after that kind of surgery. But she didn't give him a chance. She sobbed and talked, and he listened. After a while, her words blurred in his ears, but he patted her on the thigh and pretended to listen. She seemed to accept this, and he soon fell asleep.

The next night after dinner she told him she wanted to try again. He was a bit surprised but, ever hopeful, went along with her plan. And the same thing happened again. He reached orgasm almost as soon as his penis went near her vagina. This time there were no tears. Gayle tried to make a joke, and he just scowled at her. He was angry but he wasn't sure what he was angry at or why. Gayle didn't know what to do or say after her attempt at a joke. They lay there for a few minutes, and then Dave got up and went to watch TV late into the night.

Dr. Katz Explains

Early or rapid ejaculation may occur in men who have not had sex in a while, and the cause is thought to be one of lack of control of his excitement and then orgasm. It also may happen when there is fear involved, in this case fear of hurting his partner or fear that she will change her mind and stop the activity. This is not necessarily rational and there is no one to blame. It just happens.

And when it's happened once, it's more likely to happen again. This is exactly what happened the second time they tried to make love. Dave was nervous that it would happen again, so it did. This can cause distress for both the man and woman. He may withdraw, fearing that this will happen again, and he will feel humiliated. Even if the woman reassures him, he may not believe her and may then think that she is lying. This can spill over into other areas of their relationship, and he may begin to mistrust her.

From Bad to Worse

For the next few weeks, the couple moved around each other. Dave didn't want to talk about what happened, and Gayle wasn't sure what to do or say. She tried cuddling next to him while he watched TV, but then he moved away to the other chair and soon she gave up. In desperation one night, she opened a bottle of wine with dinner, and they proceeded to drink the whole bottle. Dave was quite tipsy and his mood lightened. Gayle had drunk less than he did, but she felt a little reckless and decided to take a chance. She let him brush his teeth and get into the ratty old t-shirt that he slept in, and then she put her arms around him and pushed him into their bedroom where she now slept alone.

Dave had just enough alcohol in him to forget his anger from the last two occasions when they tried to have sex. Or perhaps he was just hopeful or too full of alcohol to care. They fell onto the bed in a jumble of arms and legs and elbows and knees. Gayle almost slid onto the floor but managed to crawl back onto the bed. They were both quite breathless but it felt so good to just be careless and tipsy. But then nothing happened. Dave couldn't get an erection. This sobered him up pretty quickly, and he pulled out of Gayle's embrace and stumbled to his room, leaving Gayle alone in tears again. Why were things not working?

Dr. Katz Explains

Once a man has experienced early or rapid ejaculation, it's not uncommon for him to develop another problem, difficulty getting an erection. In Dave's case, this time it might have been the alcohol, which can cause a temporary inability to have an erection. But for Dave, even though he was a little drunk, he probably was concerned about how quickly he would ejaculate this time. Erections are, in part, caused by stimulation of the penis, but another important cause is the brain. Any fear—of failure, for example—can interfere with the nervous control of the erection, and nothing happens! This, in turn, leads to fear of failure the next time and the next.

Men often suffer great distress when they experience a problem with sex or erections. And they often keep this as a secret. They may find ways to hide it from their partner—by starting a fight if the partner starts to initiate sex or by avoiding the partner by going to bed earlier or later than the partner does. Since the development of effective erectile medications, men have been more likely to report erectile problems to their physicians.

The Morning After

The next morning, Dave entered the kitchen and didn't make eye contact with his wife. He wasn't sure if he was angry, embarrassed, or ashamed. He sure didn't know what to say or do, but he was hungry, and the kitchen was where the food was. Gayle was there, and she was feeling guilty at tricking him last night. She'd also convinced herself that this was all her fault—that if she hadn't had cancer, their life would have been everything that they planned. Now she'd ruined it. The two of them made coffee and toast in silence. He read the paper, and she polished the countertop while drinking her coffee.

After 15 minutes of this, she just couldn't keep quiet for one more moment. In a rush, the words came out . . . she was sorry, she'd ruined their life, she'd gotten him drunk because she'd thought it would help, but it didn't, and now she'd ruined everything. For once she didn't cry, and this seemed to surprise Dave, who told her calmly that she was talking nonsense, nothing was ruined, and he was going to fix things. He didn't tell her how, but he had a plan, and that plan involved getting an erectile medication from one of his friends.

Dr. Katz Explains

Kitchen scenes like this are common the morning after something has happened that's upset one or both members of a couple. Apologies and acceptance are the lubricants of married life. There has to be room for both.

Dave had thought of something that indeed might help his erectile problem, but getting medication from a friend is never a good idea. Even though these drugs are widely used and have been prescribed for millions of men, they need to be prescribed by a physician and not taken from a friend, however generous that friend is. These types of medication have side effects and should not be taken by anyone who is also taking nitrates for chest pain or by men who have a significant cardiac history. They are not available over the counter for a good reason.

A Friend Indeed

Later that week, Dave made a point of asking his friend Paul to meet for coffee. He had a plan—to get the medication from him—but he was not sure how to go about asking. He didn't want to tell Paul that he was having problems, but how else to ask? Paul had been a pharmaceutical representative before retiring, so perhaps Dave could just tell him about his problem. Paul had once joked about needing some help since he turned 65, so he should be sympathetic.

After 45 minutes of chatting about the usual stuff, Dave just came right out and asked Paul if he had one or two of the blue pills to spare. Paul kept a straight face and told him that he really would like to help, but Dave should see his physician. "No offense, pal, but I can't in good conscience give them to you. It's one of the first things we learned at the drug company: Don't give anything to your friends or family. It's just too dangerous."

Dave knew he was right and apologized for asking. But now that he'd said the words to someone else, he knew that he could talk to his doctor about it. And so he went home and made an appointment for later that week. He didn't tell Gayle what he was doing; this was his problem, and he was going to fix it.

What's a Man to Do?

That Friday, he arrived 10 minutes early for his appointment with Dr. Stinson. He had the whole conversation in his head and had practiced it over and over in the car driving to the medical center. When Dr. Stinson asked why he was there, he began to recite his speech. But he hadn't planned on Dr. Stinson interrupting and asking questions. And before he knew it, he was telling him the whole story; how he twice had an orgasm too early and how bad he felt and how now he also couldn't get an erection and he was only 62!

Dr. Stinson explained how the one thing could lead to the other, which, in turn, could make the first problem worse. Dave was amazed at how much sense that made, and he was eager to hear how he could be helped. Dr. Stinson didn't just write him a prescription for something to help the erections; he asked Dave what was the most important issue that he wanted to deal with. Dave was not sure; they were both connected, so what came first?

Dr. Stinson outlined the two options: he could take medication that would help him to get and maintain an erection. But he still might have an orgasm too quickly for his and his wife's satisfaction. Or he could take an antidepressant, which would delay orgasm. This might give him confidence, and he would not need anything to help with the erections. Dave marveled at the complexity of this. Who would have thought it was so complicated?

Dr. Katz Explains

Dave has two problems that are interacting, as Dr. Stinson clearly had seen. Dave can take medication, which helps to trap the blood in the penis by altering a complex enzyme reaction in the tissues of the penis. But that may not affect this new problem he has with early ejaculation. Part of that issue is psychological, and some sex therapy may help. But there is another potential solution that Dr. Stinson has suggested: an antidepressant taken daily that has the interesting side effect of delaying orgasm. This was discovered when people taking the medication for treatment of depression and anxiety complained that they were having difficulty achieving orgasm. This is an off-label use of the medication, meaning that it has not received U.S. Food and Drug Administration approval for the treatment of premature ejaculation.

A Man With a Plan

Dave decided that he wanted to think about this, and a voice in his head was telling him that he should talk to Gayle about it. When he thought about it, they hadn't really talked about the problem at all. They'd mostly gotten angry and not talked to each other, and Gayle had cried a lot.

But now he had some potential solutions and perhaps between the two of them, they could work things out. He was a man with a plan.

CHAPTER 16

Where to Find Help

This chapter features sources of additional information that may provide additional guidance for you. This list is not an endorsement of any of these products but rather a guide to some of what's out there.

Pamphlets

- American Association for Marriage and Family Therapy. (2002). *Female sexual problems.* Retrieved August 15, 2008, from http://www.aamft.org/families/ consumer_updates/femalesexualproblems.asp
- Silence about sexual problems can hurt relationships [JAMA Patient Page]. (1999). *JAMA, 281*(6), 584.
- National Library of Medicine. (2007). *MedlinePlus medical encyclopedia: Inhibited sexual desire.* Retrieved August 15, 2008, from http://www.nlm .nih.gov/medlineplus/ency/article/001952.htm
- The Women's Sexual Health Foundation. (2004). *Are you a woman experiencing desire difficulties?* Retrieved August 15, 2008, from http://www.twshf.org/ pdf/desire_diff_brochure_3_fold_twshf.pdf
- The Women's Sexual Health Foundation. (2004). *Talking with your doctor about sexual difficulties.* Retrieved August 15, 2008, from http://www.twshf .org/pdf/TWSHF_Talking_With_Your_Doctor.pdf

Books
Libido

- Goodwin, A.J., & Agronin, M.E. (1998). *A woman's guide to overcoming sexual fear and pain*. Oakland, CA: New Harbinger Publications.
- Reichman, J. (1998). *I'm not in the mood: What every woman should know about improving her libido*. New York: William Morrow and Company.
- Simon, J.A., & Houston, V. (2001). *Restore yourself: A woman's guide to reviving her sexual desire and passion for life*. New York: Berkley Publishing Group.
- Weiner, D.M. (2003). *The sex-starved marriage*. New York: Simon and Schuster.

Female Orgasm

- Barbach, L. (2000). *For yourself: The fulfillment of female sexuality*. New York: Anchor Books.
- Heart, M. (1998). *When the earth moves: Women and orgasm*. Berkeley, CA: Celestial Arts.
- Heiman, J., & Lopicollo, J. (1988). *Becoming orgasmic*. New York: Simon and Schuster.
- Komisaruk, B., Bayer-Flores, C., & Whipple, B. (2006). *The science of orgasm*. Baltimore: Johns Hopkins University Press.
- Paget, L. (2001). *The big O*. New York: Broadway Books.

General Sexuality

- Barbach, L. (2001). *For each other*. New York: Penguin Books.
- Brown, M., & Braveman, S. (2007). *CPR for your sex life: How to breathe life into a dead, dying, or dull sex life*. Charleston, SC: BookSurge Publishing.
- Joannides, P. (2008). *The guide to getting it on* (6th ed.). Waldport, OR: Goofy Foot Press.

Women's Sexuality

- Berman, J.R., & Berman, L.A. (2000). *For women only: A revolutionary guide to overcoming sexual dysfunction and reclaiming your sex life*. New York: Henry Holt and Company.

- Daniluk, J. (1998). *Women's sexuality across the lifespan.* New York: Guilford Press.
- Ellison, C. (2000). *Women's sexualities.* Oakland, CA: New Harbinger Publications.
- Foley, S., Kope, S.A., & Sugrue, D.P. (2002). *Sex matters for women: A complete guide to taking care of your sexual self.* New York: Guilford Press.
- Hutcherson, H. (2003). *What your mother never told you about s-e-x.* New York: Perigee Books.
- Klein, M., & Robbins, R. (1998). *Let me count the ways: Discovering great sex without intercourse.* New York: Penguin Putnam.
- Leiblum, S., & Sachs, J. (2002). *Getting the sex you want: A woman's guide to becoming proud, passionate, and pleased in bed.* New York: Crown.
- Levine, S.B. (1998). *Sexuality in mid-life.* New York: Plenum Press.

Sex and Aging

- Price, J. (2006). *Better than I ever expected.* Emeryville, CA: Seal Press.

Cancer and Sexuality

- Katz, A. (2007). *Breaking the silence on cancer and sexuality: A handbook for healthcare providers.* Pittsburgh, PA: Oncology Nursing Society.
- Schover, L. (1997). *Sexuality and fertility after cancer.* New York: John Wiley and Sons.

Web Sites

- **Cancer Survivors Network**
  www.acscsn.org
  Vast amount of information related to surviving and thriving after cancer. Sponsored by the American Cancer Society.
- **Female Sexual Dysfunction Online**
  www.femalesexualdysfunctiononline.org
  A professional Web site for clinicians and researchers. Has useful information, although academic in style.

- **Fertile Hope**
  www.fertilehope.org/index.cfm
  A nonprofit organization dedicated to providing reproductive information, support, and hope to patients with cancer and survivors whose medical treatments present the risk of infertility
- **National Sexuality Resource Center**
  www.nsrc.sfsu.edu
  Contains a wealth of information for consumers and clinicians
- **OncoLink**
  www.oncolink.com/index.cfm
  Comprehensive cancer information from the University of Pennsylvania for patients and their families
- **Out With Cancer**
  www.outwithcancer.com
  An online resource for gay, lesbian, bisexual, and transgendered people with cancer

Online Retailers

- Come as You Are (Canadian): www.comeasyouare.com
- Eve's Garden: www.evesgarden.com
- Good Vibrations: www.goodvibes.com
- The Pleasure Chest: www.apleasurechest.com
- Toys in Babeland: www.babeland.com

Professional Counseling

- The American Association of Sexuality Educators, Counselors and Therapists (www.aasect.org) has a list of qualified therapists and counselors across North America.